FAMILY HEALTH

FAMILY HEALTH

A Holistic Approach to Social Work Practice

Edited by
John T. Pardeck and Francis K. O. Yuen

AUBURN HOUSE
Westport, Connecticut • London

Library of Congress Cataloging-in-Publication Data

Family health : a holistic approach to social work practice /
edited by John T. Pardeck and Francis K. O. Yuen.
p. cm.
Includes bibliographical references and index.
ISBN 0–86569–268–8 (alk. paper)
1. Family social work. 2. Family—Health and hygiene. 3. Family—Mental health. 4. Medical social work. 5. Psychiatric social work. I. Pardeck, John T. II. Yuen, Francis K. O., date
HV697.F364 1999
362.82—dc21 98–47756

British Library Cataloguing in Publication Data is available.

Library of Congress Catalog Card Number: 98–47756
ISBN: 0–86569–268–8

First published in 1999

Auburn House, 88 Post Road West, Westport, CT 06881
An imprint of Greenwood Publishing Group, Inc.
www.greenwood.com

Printed in the United States of America

The paper used in this book complies with the Permanent Paper Standard issued by the National Information Standards Organization (Z39.48–1984).

10 9 8 7 6 5 4 3 2 1

This book is dedicated to
Mr. Kenneth C. PARDECK
and Mr. YUEN Kai Wo

Contents

Acknowledgments

Dr. Pardeck appreciates the encouragement of Jean Pardeck, Ruth Pardeck, Lois Musick, and Burl Musick. They all provided help during the preparation of this book.

Dr. Yuen is deeply indebted to his wife, Dr. Cynthia Kellen-Yuen, and their daughters, Amanda and Emily, for their support. He is obliged to his parents and siblings who have taught him the value of family.

The editors particularly appreciate the editorial assistance of Terry Brown. They would also like to express their thankfulness to the contributors for each of the chapters, the School of Social Work at Southwest Missouri State University, members of the school's Advisory Council, the students at the school, and the social workers in the region for their inspiration, encouragement, critiques, and support.

FAMILY HEALTH

1

A Family Health Approach to Social Work Practice

Francis K. O. Yuen and John T. Pardeck

Family health is an emerging practice orientation in the profession of social work. Even though the profession has always stressed the importance of the family system in practice and policy development, the concept of family health is new to the profession. Given the fact that family health is a new innovation to the field, the following serves as a guiding definition for this emerging practice approach: Family health is a state of holistic well-being of the family system. Family health is manifested by the development of, and continuous interaction among, the physical, mental, emotional, social, economic, cultural, and spiritual dimensions of the family which results in the holistic well-being of the family and its members (School of Social Work, Southwest Missouri State University, 1996).

The goal of this chapter is to develop the philosophical basis of family health and offer the theoretical underpinnings of this innovative approach to practice and policy development.

MODELS FOR DEFINING HEALTH

A family health approach to social work practice can first be understood through an analysis of the three models that have been used for defining and explaining health: the disease, illness, and sickness models. Depending on the model, the definition, treatment, and assessment tools implemented in intervention will vary greatly (Pardeck & Yuen, 1997).

The disease model is grounded in the physical aspect of a presenting problem. Disease is a biomedical concept that refers to the physiological features of nonhealth. Social workers who base their practice in a family health approach realize that the disease model has numerous limitations, especially in the assessment and treatment of mental health–related problems. Even though the disease model continues to dominate the orientation of service delivery within the mental health system, critics suggest it has a number of major limitations that include the following (Pardeck & Yuen, 1997):

1. It is grounded in the "germ theory" for explaining disease and has limited utility for assessing and treating mental illness.
2. The disease model relies on the effectiveness of differential diagnosis when there is poor reliability among those making diagnoses for mental health.
3. It seeks a single best treatment to eradicate the cause of mental illness, whereas most health-related problems have multiple causes.
4. The disease model has the potential to dehumanize clients because of its overreliance on various technologies, including computers and diagnostic tools such as the DSM-IV.
5. It has the tendency to promote authoritarian relationships between practitioners and clients in which the locus of responsibility is removed from clients.
6. The disease model acknowledges only the biological aspects of mental health and gives limited consideration of its psychosocial aspects.
7. It is a model of disease care delivery, not mental health care, and largely ignores primary prevention.

The disease model suggests that clients are viewed as passive recipients of treatment and services; as will be seen shortly, a family health approach to social work practice has a much different view of the role of clients in the assessment and treatment process.

An illness model to explaining mental health is very different from the disease model (Pardeck, 1996). An illness can exist, according to the illness model, regardless of whether a symptom is present or absent. If a client defines him- or herself as emotionally troubled, even though symptoms are not present, mental illness does exist. Subjective feelings concerning one's emotional well-being may even influence changes in the body's immune system, thus promoting the chances for physical disease to occur. Even though an illness approach to defining health has a number of strengths, social workers must also realize it has limitations. The illness approach to health focuses entirely too much on the psychological and subjective aspects of the person and disregards the important influence of the environment on individual social functioning. When using an illness approach to understanding mental health, there is also the potential to relegate professional judgment in the assessment and treatment process to a secondary level of importance (Pardeck & Yuen, 1997).

The third approach, the sickness model, is grounded in sociological theory (Pardeck, 1996). This approach emerged from the writings of Talcott Parsons (1951), who suggested one's level of healthiness as being a label created by society. The process of defining a person as sick occurs regardless of whether an illness is present or absent. Interpreting health through such a process has a number of obvious limitations. Specifically, the subjective nature of health is not important when viewing health from a sickness model. Furthermore, the environment is emphasized to such a degree in the sickness model that the psychological aspects of health are disregarded. Keeping these limitations in mind, the sickness model includes the following theoretical principles (Pardeck & Yuen, 1997). The sick person:

1. Is not held responsible for confronting his or her condition and cannot get better by an act of self-motivation.
2. Has a right to some exemptions from normal social activities based on the severity and nature of his or her illness.
3. Does not like being ill and wants to get well.
4. Must seek competent professional help in order to improve health.

Salvador Minuchin (1974) concludes that much of one's ability to cope with sickness is affected by one's ability to adapt to his or her social environment. The family system plays an important role in this

Table 1.1
Approaches for Defining and Understanding Health

	Disease Model	Illness Model	Sickness Model	Family Health Perspective
Basis	Biomedical	Psychological	Sociological	Biopsychosocial/ Ecological
Orientation	Pathological symptoms	Subjective Perception	Socially constructed	Ecological and family systems
Assessment and Intervention	Professional objective diagnosis of symptoms	Professional evaluations and understanding of one's self-constructed conditions	Professional assessments of psychosocial environment	Professional interventions based on the dynamics of people's subjective perspectives and changing their social environment

adaptation process. A family health approach to practice recognizes the importance of Parsons's and Minuchin's work; however, a family health perspective is far more than simply helping clients adapt to their social milieu. Family health stresses that social workers must be involved in strategies aimed at changing the social environment of clients. These strategies include advocacy, empowerment, policy development, and implementation (Pardeck & Yuen, 1997).

The family system is an important component of Parsons's (1951) and Minuchin's (1974) health perspectives. Both social theorists clearly recognize that a supportive social environment will have positive effects on the health of individuals and their family systems (Pardeck, 1996). Social environments that are not supportive will result in poor adaptation for individuals and their families (Pardeck, 1996).

Of the three models explaining the origins of health, the disease model appears to have the greatest limitations. The disease model views clients as passive recipients of the assessment and treatment process and almost totally disregards the social environment. The family health approach to social work practice suggests that the environment plays a critical role in a client's social functioning. Furthermore, the disease model also does not include the subjective nature of health. Of the three models covered, the illness model provides solid grounding for the family health approach to social work practice (Pardeck & Yuen, 1997).

Table 1.1 offers the basis, orientation, and assessment and intervention aspects of the disease, illness, and sickness models (Pardeck & Yuen, 1997). Also included in table 1.1 is the family health approach to social work practice. As seen in table 1.1 the disease model has limited utility for the family health approach to practice because it does not consider the importance of the social environment on the family system. Even though the social environment is a critical component to explaining health from a sickness model, it has limitations because it does not focus on the role that the individual plays in shaping his or her environment. The illness model to health stresses the role the individual plays in shaping one's subjective interpretation of health. The client's subjective interpretation to defining one's level of health is a critical aspect of a family health approach to social work practice. Most importantly, such an approach stresses one's total well-being as significantly influenced by the family system and the larger social ecology (Pardeck & Yuen, 1997).

SYSTEMS THEORY

A system can be viewed as a whole made up of individual parts. When change occurs in one part, the other parts of the system are affected. Systems theory focuses on linkages and relationships that connect individuals with each other such as those found in the family system (Pardeck & Yuen, 1997).

Systems theory provides a paradigm that focuses on multiple levels of phenomena simultaneously and emphasizes the interaction and transaction between parts. This theory helps social workers understand behavior in context and illustrates how systems impact individual social functioning. At a conceptual level, systems can be understood as open or closed. Healthy systems are typically open; closed systems are generally dysfunctional. This is a basic premise guiding a family health approach to practice (Pardeck & Yuen, 1997).

Open systems are those that exchange matter and energy with their environments. For example, a lighted candle that is covered with a glass jar is similar to a closed system because it lacks a source of oxygen and gradually goes out. When the glass jar is removed and the candle is relit, the lighted candle exchanges oxygen and carbon dioxide with the atmosphere; it is then similar to an open system (Pardeck & Yuen, 1997).

Systems theory suggests that all systems attempt to maintain a steady state as they transact with their social environments. Furthermore, systems are self-regulating. There is a tendency for systems to seek equilibrium even after the larger social ecology changes. This can result in a functional or dysfunctional system. For example, a family living in a community that is in transition toward crime and poverty will ultimately be affected. If the family is a healthy system, it will attempt to maintain this steady state regardless of the larger dysfunctional social environment. A family health approach to social work practice attempts to help families define, develop, and maintain healthy states and change nonsupportive social environments through micro- and macrolevel interventions (Pardeck & Yuen, 1997).

The exchange process occurring between a system and its social environment is referred to as input and output. The resources used by a system to obtain its goals are called input. Likewise, output refers to the products created by systems after all input has been processed. This exchange process occurring in all systems is a vital concept underpinning a family health approach to social work practice (Pardeck & Yuen, 1997).

Through the input/output process, social workers realize the delicate balance between the family system and the larger community. The community must provide families with quality schools and social and economic supports in order for families to operate at an optimal level. If this kind of input is not forthcoming from the community, families will not contribute positive output in exchange. What emerges is a family system that gradually becomes a closed system which may be characterized by abuse, neglect, and other kinds of dysfunctional behaviors. Thus the practitioner realizes that healthy families often thrive in healthy communities. Disorganized communities create an environment that has a negative impact on family health (Pardeck & Yuen, 1997).

A family health perspective views communities as a critical human association that supports the family system. These associations are based on ties of kinship, relationship, and shared experiences in which individuals voluntarily attempt to provide meaning in their lives, meet individual needs, and accomplish personal goals (Brueggeman, 1996). Communities are social systems that may take on various forms including churches and temples, ethnic and cultural organizations, neighborhoods, or families. Social workers grounded in a family health approach to practice should be cognizant of the interrelatedness of clients' well-being and the state of the larger community. For example, newly arrived refugees and immigrants often rely on their ethnic/cultural communities or religious organizations as critical support systems to assist in establishing themselves in a new country. These communities provide the communal ties that enable newcomers to transcend and meet the challenges of a strange and sometimes hostile environment (Pardeck & Yuen, 1997).

Another important concept in systems theory is equifinality, which means similar results can be obtained from different kinds of beginning points. For example, two infants, one born prematurely and the other at full term, will look very different at birth; however, if they are both provided appropriate care, the differences will disappear as they move through the life cycle. Even though the children's initial state was very different, human beings attain similar states of physical growth and development if properly supported (Pardeck, 1996).

Systems theory is an excellent strategy for providing insight into the interrelationship and interconnectedness among human beings. Furthermore, systems theory provides important insight into the family system for social workers grounded in a family health approach to practice (Pardeck & Yuen, 1997).

Michael P. Nichols and Richard C. Schwartz (1991) identified a number of basic tenets of systems theory that can be applied to understanding family functioning and health. These tenets are important to practitioners using a family health approach to practice because they provide a holistic orientation to the assessment and treatment of the family system (Pardeck & Yuen, 1997).

First, systems theory suggests that the whole is more than the sum of its parts. In relation to the family system, the family is more than just individual family members. The nature of the transaction and interaction between family members, the rules that govern these processes, and their repetitive patterns must be considered to gain insight into family functioning. Furthermore, the structural organization within the family is an important aspect of family functioning. Given the importance of the family system on the social functioning of the individual, it is an important target of social intervention in practice.

Second, a family systems approach places great emphasis on the contextual elements within the family system and the influence the larger society has on individual family members. These elements are often the target of family intervention at both the micro- and macrolevels of interventions (Pardeck & Yuen, 1997).

Third, the concept of homeostasis is critical to understanding the family system. The homeostatic process occurs when the family system responds to internal and environmental pressures. In particular, the homeostatic function of the symptom as reflected through the identified client in protecting the system is critical to intervention (Pardeck & Yuen, 1997).

Fourth, the concept of circular causality is fundamental to understanding the family system. Traditional models of treatment are based on linear causality. A systems approach stresses the reciprocal, interactional, and transactional pattern of behaviors that influence family functioning (Pardeck & Yuen, 1997).

Circular causality can be understood in a certain sense as a new epistemology in Western thought; however, it has been a dominant orientation of time and causality for many cultural groups. Florence R. Kluckhohn and Fred L. Strodtbeck (1961) and Edwin J. Nichols (1987) in their work describe the spiral and present orientation of Hispanic and African populations and the circular and past orientation of Asian populations.

Fifth, the family life cycle, an important component of the family health approach to practice, is a predictable pattern through which all families evolve. Depending on the strengths of the family system, this movement through the life cycle, later referred to as life course, can go smoothly or be stressful (Pardeck & Yuen, 1997).

The above points provide insight into understanding, assessing, and treating families through a family health approach to social work practice. They clearly suggest that individual social functioning is connected to the functioning of the family system. The family health approach to practice is grounded in the notion that the individual is best understood within the context of the family system.

THE FAMILY LIFE CYCLE

The early work by Evelyn R. Duvall (1955) was built on the assumption that all families moved through predictable series of stages. Out of this early work the term *family life cycle* emerged. Elizabeth Carter and Monica McGoldrick (1988, p. 15), building on the work of Duvall, defined the family life cycle as follows:

Stage 1. Leaving home: single young adults.

Stage 2. The joining of families through marriage: the new couple.

Stage 3. Families with young children.

Stage 4. Families with adolescents.

Stage 5. Launching children and moving on.

Stage 6. Families in later life.

However, family theorists have begun to realize that families do not necessarily move through an orderly family life cycle. Only a small percentage of families actually move through the life cycle as defined by Carter and McGoldrick (1988). The majority of families experience nondevelopmental events that influence how they develop.

As family theorists now realize the unpredictability of family life, they suggest the term *life course* versus *life cycle* better describes family development. Life course implies that development is like traveling along a highway that has many intersections: Each intersection is a transition where one route is taken and others are not. The route taken determines the life course of the family system. The events provide evidence for the many possibilities that may well influence the life course of families (Burr, Day, & Bahr, 1993):

1. Nearly 50% of American families end their first marriages in divorce.
2. Roughly 15% of families never have children.
3. About 20% of Americans have more than one divorce.
4. Many people remarry and create blended families.

These numerous possible family events suggest great potential for variability in the life cycle of families and the individuals who compose family systems. Just as there are different family forms, there is also great variation in family development. Even so, there continue to be some predictable events indicative of family life. Courtship usually precedes weddings, and births normally precede childrearing. One's aging typically comes late in the family development; however, coping with the aging of one's parents and grandparents comes earlier. Midlife crises normally happen in one's forties and fifties; these life events have an impact on family development. Even though families take various routes during their development, there are life events that can help social work practitioners intervene more effectively with family systems. The social worker grounded in the family health approach to practice needs to be knowledgeable of the life events that affect family development (Burr et al., 1993).

FAMILY HEALTH AND THE ECOLOGICAL APPROACH

Social workers grounded in a family health approach to practice are sensitive to the clients' worldview and the ecological context in which they function. An ecological view is critical to a family health approach to practice because it stresses the reciprocal, transactional, and holistic dynamics that exist between the person and the environment. Carel B. Germain and Alex Gitterman (1987) identified the major concepts of the ecological perspective: reciprocal causality/exchange, adaptedness, life stress, coping, niche, habitat, and relatedness. The ecological perspective concludes that neither persons nor their environment can be fully understood except in relation to each other (Pardeck & Yuen, 1997).

Ecological theory is prescriptive in that it offers intervention strategies at both the micro- and macrolevels. The ecological perspective provides strategies for helping social workers impact client systems through policy and planning activities as well as through therapeutic and other microlevel interventions. From a family health approach to social work practice, the most important client system the practitioner works with is the family system (Pardeck & Yuen, 1997).

The ecological approach provides strategies that help social workers address problems and needs at various systemic levels including the individual, family, and larger community. An ecological perspective offers strategies for helping social workers shift from a therapeutic role to a policy and planning role within a broad theoretical context (Pardeck & Yuen, 1997).

Six distinct professional roles are found within the ecological approach to social work intervention. These roles complement a family health approach to practice because they offer effective strategies for working with the family system. These roles include (Pardeck, 1996):

1. *Conferee*: Derived from the idea of conference, this role focuses on actions that are taken when the social worker serves as the primary source of assistance to the client in problem solving.
2. *Enabler*: The enabler role focuses on actions taken when the social worker structures, arranges, and manipulates events, interactions, and environmental variables to facilitate and enhance system functioning.
3. *Broker*: This role is defined as actions taken when the social worker's objective is to link the consumer with goods and services or to control their quality.
4. *Mediator*: This role focuses on actions taken when the social worker's objective is to reconcile opposing or disparate points of view and bring people together in united actions.

5. *Advocate*: This role is defined as actions taken when the social worker secures services or resources on behalf of the client in the face of identified resistance or develops resources or services in cases where they are inadequate or nonexistent.
6. *Guardian*: The role of guardian is defined as actions taken when the social worker performs a social control function or takes protective action when the client's competency level is deemed inadequate.

There is a blurring of roles when a social worker uses an ecological approach to practice. For example, the roles of conferee and enabler are difficult to separate. When social workers implement the broker role, they also may find themselves enabling and advocating. The complementarity among the roles should be noted, as well as their tendency to cluster rather than remain distinct. This is a significant departure from the traditional specialization approaches often used in social work practice. The social worker using a family health perspective has the knowledge and skills to work at multiple levels of the social ecology (Pardeck & Yuen, 1997).

SOCIAL CONSTRUCTIONIST AND POSTMODERN PERSPECTIVES

Systems theory and the ecological perspective are important theoretical frameworks for family health social work practice. Social workers should, however, realize that both approaches have limitations. One important limitation is that both theories have a tendency to deemphasize individual volition (Brueggeman, 1996). Furthermore, there is too much emphasis placed on the adaptation of clients to their social environment rather than changing it. These limitations must be considered by practitioners when working with clients.

Knowledge of the work of social constructionists may help practitioners understand the potential limitations of the systems and ecological approaches to practice. Social constructionists emphasize that people have the ability to make sense of their experiences and give meaning to them. "Experiences of the objective and the subjective realms are selectively arranged on the basis of assumed themes, which organize, structure, and give meaningfulness to the person or family" (Kilpatrick & Holland, 1995, p. 25). The family health approach stresses the importance of considering the client's and his or her family system's view of social reality when assessing a presenting problem.

Social workers implementing a family health perspective provide services to persons and their families at multiple levels. These services are designed to promote family health; they should not only be meaningful to the clients and their family systems but also facilitate total well-being of family members. Clients and their family systems must be active participants in the helping process when social work practice is conducted through a family health approach.

Another theory related to social constructionism is postmodernism. Postmodernism celebrates diversity and suggests that reality is largely shaped by each individual's experience. What this means is there is no ultimate "objective reality"; reality is situational and family and community based. For example, what it means to be poor, homeless, an old person, or a person with a disability is largely defined by persons experiencing each of these personal situations; reality for each situation is defined by the person and shaped by other social systems such as the family and community (Fisher, 1991). Practitioners must be sensitive to these definitions in order to conduct appropriate assessments and interventions (Murphy & Pardeck, 1998).

What is powerful about a postmodern approach to social work practice is that it demystifies traditional theories and limits their authority in defining social problems and social reality. As suggested by postmodernism, accepted social scientific theories are often an extension of a dominant group's self-interests and ideologies. Typically, the social realities experienced by oppressed groups are greatly different than those of dominant groups. A postmodern view suggests that the perceptions of social problems and social reality as defined by all groups are equally relevant for understanding the social world (Murphy & Pardeck, 1998).

A postmodern view suggests there is not an ultimate authoritative source of knowledge. For example, empirically based research is treated with the same respect as other sources of knowledge. A postmodern view concludes that knowledge is constructed through language and that facts are embedded within language. Social workers must be sensitive to these notions when conducting assessments and intervention. In other words, social work intervention must be truly "community based." Like the constructionists' view, the postmodern perspective offers social workers a very important worldview for assessing and treating family systems. Social workers grounded in the family health approach to practice should be aware of the constructionist and postmodern perspectives that provide new insights into social problems and social reality (Murphy & Pardeck, 1998).

FAMILY HEALTH AND SOCIAL WORK INTERVENTION

Family health as an area of practice represents a distinct departure from the traditional disease model that has dominated the fields of medicine and mental health. Even though the field of family health is new to social work practice, the seminal work on family systems theory has its roots in the traditions of social work. Given the traditional emphasis placed on the family system within the profession, the following basic premises are offered as a general orientation to family health as an approach to social work practice (Pardeck & Yuen, 1997):

1. Family health is based on a psychosocial orientation to understanding individual social functioning. The traditional disease model assumes pathology can be reduced to measurable biological variables; this view is inconsistent with the family health perspective. Even though the disease model has been very successful in treating numerous diseases, especially infectious diseases, the disease model has not been very successful in dealing with the numerous social problems confronting clients who seek social work services. In fact, M. A. Baird and William J. Doherty (1990) have noted, ''Focusing only on the biological level represents a cultural bias disguised as scientific theory'' (p. 397).

The psychosocial perspective places confronting problems of clients and their families within a larger social context involving social systems. In order to treat presenting problems, the social worker grounded in the family health approach to practice must attend not only to biological factors but also to the person, family, community, and social context of the person-in-the-environment. The focus of intervention thus becomes the interaction and transaction of the family system within the larger social ecology. The locus of the family health approach to social work practice is not the deficits or disease of the individual but rather the promotion and maintenance of the total well-being of the individual in his or her family (Pardeck & Yuen, 1997).

2. Family health social work practice focuses on the family as the most important context within which problems occur. A family health approach to social work practice stresses not only the biopsychosocial model but also the family level or context within which problems occur. Four key concepts are critical to this perspective (Pardeck & Yuen, 1997).

First, the family is a primary source of many beliefs about health and behavior. The work of Minuchin (1974) has developed a direct linkage between physical illness and family functioning. Specifically, family systems characterized as enmeshed, overprotective, and rigid often foster psychosomatic physical illness. Even though recent research by J. C. Coyne and B. J. Anderson (1988) has challenged this position, few would argue that the family does not play a central role in the social and physical well-being of family members. Lois V. Pratt (1976) has identified characteristics of the "energized family" thought to be resistant to the development of illness. These characteristics include positive family interaction, established community ties, encouragement of autonomy, creative problem solving based on open communication, and the ability to adjust to the changing life events of the family system. Finally, many behaviors related to health are developed within the context of the family system, including smoking, diet, and exercise (Baird & Doherty, 1990). It is important, however, to note that the energized family in different cultures may have very different characteristics (Pardeck & Yuen, 1997).

Second, the stress families often feel when going through the family life course can be manifested in social and physical symptoms. These life events include marriage, birth of a child, adolescence, leaving home, midlife crisis, death of a family member, and retirement (Carter & McGoldrick, 1988). Thomas L. Campbell (1986) reports research that illustrates the relationship between stressful life events and increased illness.

Third, problems in psychological and social functioning can serve as an adaptive function for the family and can be maintained by family patterns. Psychological problems can be understood as a barometer of the stress currently being felt within a family system. Social workers, for example, often view alcoholism as a presenting problem that maintains the homeostasis of a dysfunctional family system. A child's abdominal pain may also stabilize conflictual marital relations by keeping the parents focused on the child and not the marital problems. In other words, getting well can threaten the homeostasis of the family system; family members thus encourage the troubled family member to maintain his or her sick role (Pardeck & Yuen, 1997).

Fourth, families are a powerful resource when members are confronted with problems. The social worker grounded in a family health approach assesses and intervenes with family members in the context of the family system. The social worker and the family collaborate in the development and implementation of intervention for the entire family system (Pardeck & Yuen, 1997).

3. A family health approach to social work practice requires collaboration between the social worker and allied professionals. The effective social worker realizes that he or she cannot meet all the needs of a family system under pressure. Many problems confronting family systems require the help of other professionals. It is critical for the social worker grounded in a family health approach to practice developing good relationships with physicians, psychologists, and other professionals. A family health approach to social work practice uses a holistic orientation to assessment and intervention; thus, the approach can only be successful with the help of other supportive professionals (Pardeck & Yuen, 1997).

4. Social workers using a family health approach view themselves as "a part of" rather than "apart from" the intervention process. The disease model approach to treating mental health problems, for example, views the practitioner as an objective outsider who assesses, diagnoses, and treats problems. This approach does not consider how the practitioner may influence and be influenced by a client's behavior. When intervention does not go well, a practitioner grounded in a disease model may blame the client and label him or her as "noncompliant." A family health approach to practice encourages social workers to observe their interaction with clients and reflect on how their behavior contributes as much to what transpires as their clients' transactions with them. This interactional and reflective process enables social workers to become more responsive and sensitive to the needs of clients and their families from diverse backgrounds (Pardeck & Yuen, 1997).

These premises form the basis upon which a family health approach to social work practice is conducted (Pardeck & Yuen, 1997). The research on family systems clearly supports the validity and effectiveness of the family health approach to social work practice; this research is reviewed in chapter 2.

REFERENCES

Baird, M. A., & Doherty, W. J. (1990). Risks and benefits of a family systems approach to medical care. *Family Medicine, 22*, 396–403.

Brueggeman, W. (1996). *The practice of macro social work.* Chicago: Nelson Hall.

Burr, W. R., Day, R. D., & Bahr, S. B. (1993). *Family science.* Pacific Grove, CA: Brooks/Cole.

Campbell, T. L. (1986). The family's impact on health: A critical review and annotated bibliography. *Family Systems Medicine, 4*, 135–328.

Carter, E. A., & McGoldrick, M. (Eds.). (1988). *The changing family life cycle: A framework for family therapy.* New York: Gardner Press.

Coyne, J. C., & Anderson, B. J. (1988). Psychosomatic family reconsidered: Diabetes in context. *Journal of Marital and Family Therapy, 14*, 113–123.

Duvall, E. (1955). *Family development.* New York: J. B. Lippincott.

Fisher, D. D. V. (1991). *An introduction to constructivism for social workers.* New York: Praeger.

Germain, C. B., & Gitterman, A. (1987). Ecological perspective. In A. Minahan (Ed.), *Encyclopedia of social work* (18th ed., pp. 488–499). Silver Spring, MD: National Association of Social Workers.

Kilpatrick, A., & Holland, T. (1995). *Working with families.* Needham Heights, MA: Allyn and Bacon.

Kluckhohn, F., & Strodtbeck, F. (1961). *Variations in value orientations.* Evanston, IL: Row, Peterson.

Minuchin, S. (1974). *Families and family therapy.* Cambridge, MA: Harvard University Press.

Murphy, J. W., & Pardeck, J. T. (1998). Renewing social work practice through a postmodern perspective. In R. G. Meinert, J. T. Pardeck, & J. W. Murphy (Eds.), *Postmodernism, religion, and the future of social work* (pp. 5–19). New York: Haworth Press.

Nichols, E. (1987, September 11). *The philosophical aspects of cultural difference.* Presented at the First Annual National Association of Social Workers Conference, New Orleans, LA.

Nichols, M. P., & Schwartz, R. C. (1991). *Family therapy: Concepts and methods* (2nd ed.). Needham Heights, MA: Allyn and Bacon.

Pardeck, J. T. (1996). *Social work practice: An ecological approach.* Westport, CT: Auburn House.

Pardeck, J. T., & Yuen, F. K. O. (1997). A family health approach to social work practice. *Family Therapy, 24*, 115–128.

Parsons, T. (1951). *The social system.* New York: Free Press.

Pratt, L. (1976). *Family structure and effective health behavior: The energized family.* Boston: Houghton-Mifflin.

School of Social Work, Southwest Missouri State University. (1996). *A working paper on family health.* Springfield, MO: Author.

2

The Properties of the Family Health Approach

Francis K. O. Yuen

Family health is an approach or practice model that includes a set of theoretical orientations and skills. It is a state of holistic well-being of the family system. Family health is manifested by the development of, and continuous interaction among, the physical, mental, emotional, social, economic, cultural, and spiritual dimensions of the family which results in the holistic well-being of the family and its members (School of Social Work, Southwest Missouri State University, 1996).

As the family health approach is being utilized as a social work approach, it may be necessary to differentiate it from closely related terms such as paradigm, theory, practice model, method, skill, technique, and technology. Carel B. Germain cites Thomas S. Kuhn's 1962 definition of paradigm as "a structure of law, theory, applications, and instrumentation from which coherent research traditions spring." In essence, a paradigm provides an overall way to understand and interpret phenomena presented. It affects the direction and process of the inquiry. However, Kuhn also believes that "behavioral sciences have not yet developed paradigms, so a professional practice based on these sciences must also be in a preparadigmatic state" (cited in Germain, 1983, p. 49).

Theory has been used to refer to conceptualizations, prescriptions for behavior, or untested ideas (Reynolds, 1971). William Wiersma (1969) defines theory as "a generalization or a series of generalizations by which we attempt to explain some phenomena in some systematic manner" (p. 11). Essentially, a theory is a set of interrelated propositions or concepts, organized in some systematic manner, that offers an explanation of some phenomena.

Germain (1983, p. 31) further clarifies the definitions of several often confusing terms: approach, practice model, method, skill, technique, and technology. "Approach refers to recognizable or recognized perspective entities often called practice models." To distinguish between the theoretical model in science and the practice model in social science, a theoretical model has the ability and utility of prediction while a practice model "merely sets forth the several dimensions of a coherent, consistent approach to social work practice but has no predictive value." Method refers to designated "practice activities with a particular size unit," such as casework, group work, and community work. Skill refers to a "particular area of practitioner action, such as observation, engagement, data collection, assessment, contracting, setting goals and planning, and achieving goals. Technique is used to designate a more specific procedure within such an area of skill." Approaches, methods, skills, and techniques make up technology.

THE TECHNOLOGY OF FAMILY HEALTH

Technology is a professional values-guided application of theories, knowledge, and skills to practice (Germain, 1983). The theoretical orientations of the family health approach include the systems theory, ecological perspectives, social constructivist perspective, developmental theories, and other relevant family theories. Figure 2.1 illustrates the context and relationships among the different components of the technology of a family health–centered social work approach. The systems theory and ecological perspectives provide the context in which transactions between individuals and their environments take place. Social constructivist perspectives and developmental theories allow the subjective meaning and the reality of growth and change to be considered in the transactions. The editors discussed details of the theoretical orientations of the family health approach in the previous chapter of this book.

Individual and family as habitats occupy particular niches in the environment; their existence and reciprocal exchanges with others form the relatedness as well as the life experience of rewards and difficulties. Individual and family develop particular coping strategies, meaningful to

Figure 2.1
Theoretical Orientations for Family Health Approach

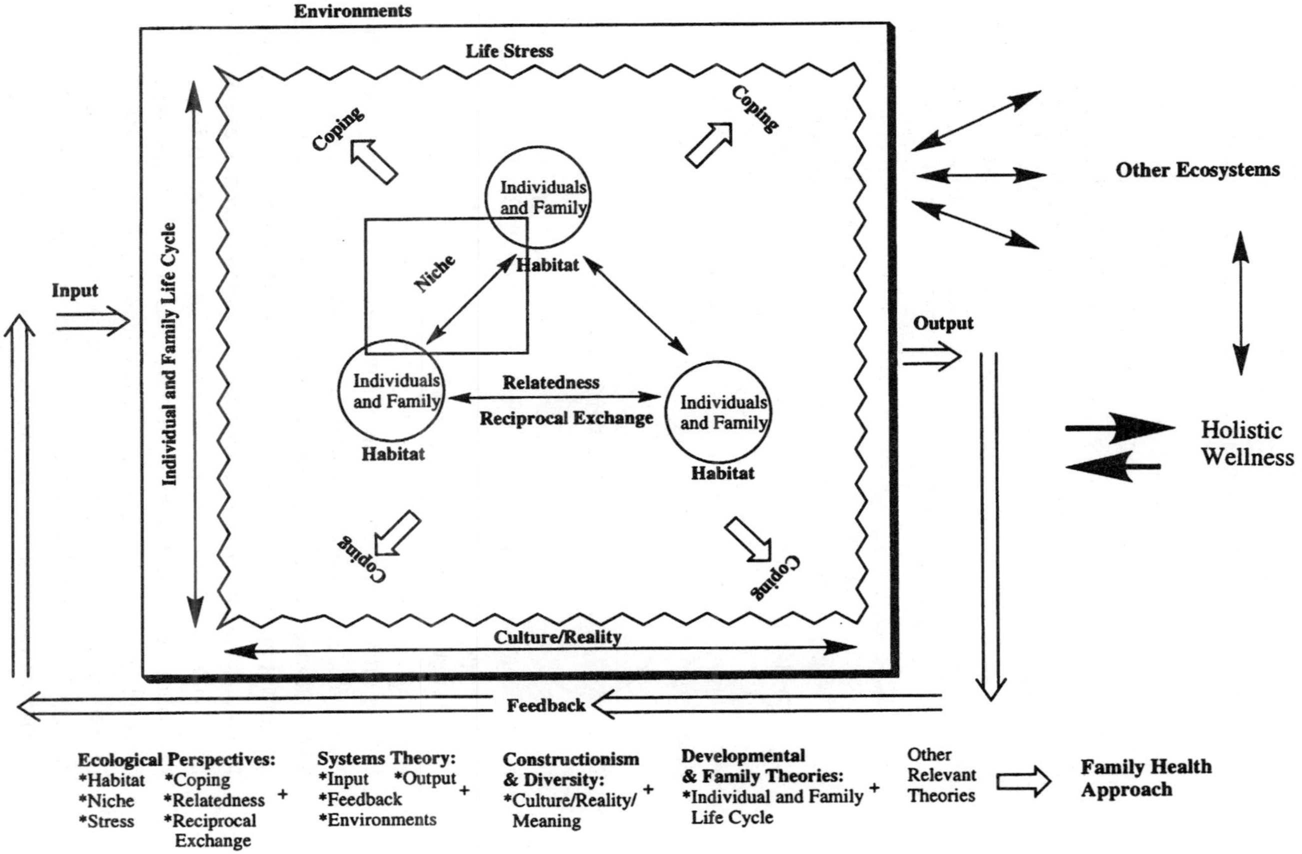

Figure 2.2
Family Health Approach and the Knowledge Development of Social Work

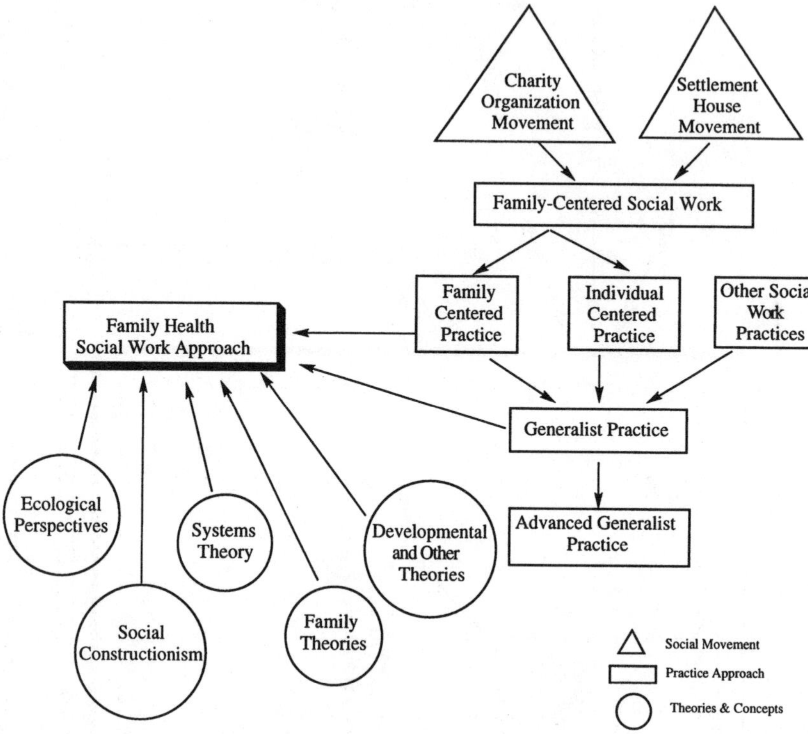

their culture and reality, to deal with various life stresses throughout the individual and family life cycles. The environments in which they reside behave either as closed systems that will eventually become extinct or as open systems that require continuous input, output, and feedback to thrive. These environments also interact and network constantly with other ecosystems. Family health–centered social work practitioners have the ability to understand the dynamics of these networks and are able to provide proper interventions. The goals of their interventions are to restore, maintain, or achieve the holistic wellness of the individual and the family.

The family health approach draws from existing knowledge and skills in the social work profession as well as those from related disciplines. Although it emphasizes the holistic and strength-oriented perspectives toward family well-being, the approach recognizes the importance of therapeutic treatments for illness and sickness. Figure 2.2 explains how the family health approach relates to knowledge development in social work. Expanding on Germain's figure (1983, p. 30) on the development of family-centered social work, figure 2.2 illustrates how the family health approach is a further development of family-centered practice and is related to, but different from, generalist practice.

According to Germain (1983), family-centered practice evolves from the Charity Organization Society and the Settlement House movements. It further becomes individual-centered practice (i.e., diagnostic and functional schools) and family-centered practice. As generalist practice is adopted by the profession (see further discussions) to conceptualize the social work profession, advanced generalist practice is being considered as the extension of the generalist approach. Although the family health approach is associated with the family-centered practice orientation, it also draws from the philosophy and intervention skills of generalist practice. With an organized blending of knowledge and skills from ecological perspectives, system theory, social constructivism, and developmental and family theories, the family health approach attempts to provide a family well-being focused practice model for social work practice.

John Pardeck, Francis Yuen, Jim Daley, and Catherine Hawkins (1998) identify the family health intervention skills that include: (a) developmental assessment, (b) resource linkage, (c) supportive intervention, (d) confrontive intervention, (e) empowering framework, (f) using social learning approaches, (g) recognizing the level of prevention and readiness for change, (h) utilization of the family unit as change agent, and (i) understanding and assessing the construction of a client's reality. Daley and Hawkins further discuss the intervention issues for family health approach in the following chapter of this book.

John T. Pardeck (1996) and Pardeck and Francis K. O. Yuen (1997) list six ecological practice roles that complement a family health approach to practice because they offer effective strategies for working with families:

1. *Conferee*: Derived from the idea of conference, the conferee role focuses on actions that are taken when the practitioner serves as the primary source of assistance to the client in problem solving.
2. *Enabler*: The enabler role focuses on actions taken when the practitioner structures, arranges, and manipulates events, interactions, and environmental variables to facilitate and enhance system functioning.

3. *Broker*: The role of broker is defined as actions taken when the practitioner's objective is to link the consumer with goods and services or control the quality of those goods and services.

4. *Mediator*: The mediator role focuses on actions taken when the practitioner's objective is to reconcile opposing or disparate points of view and bring the "contestants" together in united actions.

5. *Advocate*: The role of advocate is defined as actions taken when the practitioner secures services or resources on behalf of the client in the face of identified resistance or develops resources or services in cases where they are inadequate or nonexistent.

6. *Guardian*: The guardian role is defined as actions taken when the practitioner performs in a social control function or takes protective action when the client's competency level is deemed inadequate.

There is a blurring of roles when a practitioner uses an ecological approach to practice. For example, the roles of conferee and enabler at times are difficult to separate. When practitioners implement the broker role, they also may find themselves enabling and advocating. The complementarity among the above roles should be noted, as well as their tendency to cluster rather than remain distinct. This approach is a significant departure from the traditional specialization approaches often used in social work practice. The practitioner using a family health perspective has the knowledge and skills to work in multilevels of the social ecology (Pardeck, 1996).

CONTRASTING FAMILY HEALTH, GENERALIST, AND ADVANCED GENERALIST APPROACHES

The family health approach utilizes some generalist practice knowledge and skills such as the multilevel and multimethod intervention as its foundation knowledge, but it has a very specific orientation to family well-being. Pardeck and associates (1998, pp. 34–36) detail the differences between the family health, generalist, and advanced generalist approaches.

Generalist Approaches

In 1984, the Council of Social Work Education (CSWE) adopted generalist practice as the standard for undergraduate social work education. It is expected that generalist practice would serve as a ''unifying conceptualization for the total profession'' (Landon, 1995, p. 1101). However,

> there is no agreed-upon definition of generalist practice, and CSWE has stated that all programs will proffer their own definitions and rationale. . . . (the primary commonalties were) the centrality of the multimethod and multilevel approaches, based on an eclectic choice of theory base and the necessity for incorporating the dual vision of the profession on private issues and social justice concerns. (1995, pp. 1102–1103)

Patty Gibbs, Barry Locke, and Roger Lohmann (1990) acknowledge the lack of ''agreement on what is meant by 'generalist' and, in particular, 'advanced generalist' practice and education has remained problematic over the years'' (p. 234). They cite ''problem-solving centered rather than methods-driven'' and ''uses the person-in-environment configuration for assessment and intervention, giving practice a holistic emphasis throughout the entire problem-solving process'' (pp. 234–235) as the two major feature of generalist practice approach.

Louise C. Johnson (1995) describes the multimethod, multilevel, eclectic nature of generalist practice. ''This is, in essence, the meaning of generalist practice. In developing a plan, the focal system for change may be any system experiencing a lack of need fulfillment or contributing to the lack of need fulfillment. The change strategy is chosen from a repertoire or group of strategies that the generalist worker possesses. This repertoire contains strategies appropriate for work with a variety of systems (individuals, families, small groups, agencies, and communities)'' (p. 13). Karen Kirst-Ashman and Grafton H. Hull (1997) provide a similar assertion. They define generalist practice as ''the application of an eclectic knowledge base, professional values, and a wide range of skills to target any system size for change within the context of three primary processes. First, generalist practice involves working effectively within an organizational structure and doing so under supervision. Second, it requires the assumption of a wide range of professional roles.

Third, generalist practice involves the application of critical thinking skills to the problem-solving process'' (pp. 7–8).

''A multi-method, multi-level approach drawing from a vast repertoire of skills and including the ability to target any client system whether at micro, mezzo or macro level'' (Pardeck et al., 1998, p. 32) are the common themes for generalist approach. Consequently, one of the drawbacks for this general, universal, and all-inclusive nature of generalist is that there is no boundary.

Advanced Generalist Approaches

In 1988, CSWE adopted advanced generalist as one of five possible areas of specialty in graduate social work education. Gibbs and associates (1990) believe there is an educational progression from generalist to advanced generalist. On both the bachelor of social work (BSW) and master of social work (MSW) levels, generalists and advanced generalists perform similar roles including broker, advocate, evaluator, outreach worker, teacher, behavior changer, consultant, caregiver, data manager, administrator, enabler, mediator, and community planner. The difference between them is that ''advanced generalist practice is defined less by the unique roles performed by MSWs than by the expectations of greater depth and breadth of performance . . . and the capacity for independent practice'' (Gibbs et al., 1990, p. 236). Mona S. Schatz, Lowell E. Jenkins, and Braford W. Sheafor (1990) surveyed educators and practitioners and found their expectation of advanced generalists was that they would apply generalist skills into ''greater depth and in relation to more complex and technical issues'' (Landon, 1995, p. 1105).

Advanced generalists therefore are expected to have more exposure to the generalist principle and be more independent and capable of dealing with more complex practice situations. Pardeck and associates (1998) conclude that ''the boundary of where generalist stops and advanced generalist starts is not defined. The MSW graduate theoretically has the same framework of skills as the undergraduate social work graduate. They just have more exposure to how the generalist model can be used in more complex settings'' (p. 33).

Comparison of Generalist, Advanced Generalist, and Family Health Approaches

Basically, the family health–centered social work practitioner has a multimethod, multilevel, problem-oriented philosophy consistent with a generalist approach. It is expected that these practitioners can use such skills as broker or advocate. What is needed is a deeper understanding of the family as a focal point of intervention and strategies for enhancing physical or emotional health.

''The generalist model seeks to build a basic understanding of person-in-environment context for social work practice (micro, mezzo, and macro) and the application of different methods (e.g., enabler, advocate, change agent, administrator) to any setting where the social worker is employed. There is no central theory or focus. In fact, there is a strong emphasis on not having a central focus, rather to maximize flexibility and role definition'' (Pardeck et al., 1998).

The family health approach employs the generalist multimethods and multilevels intervention skills. With the clear and well-defined family health orientation and expertise, practitioners place the well-being of the family at the center of their interventions. They are prepared to provide holistic interventions to the clients, supported by current literature and research. These interventions are also sensible and meaningful to both the clients and the practitioners. Table 2.1 provides comparisons among the generalist, advanced generalist, and family health approach practices (Pardeck, et al., 1998, 35).

Although detailed family health intervention skill issues will be discussed in the following chapters, several major categories were identified by Pardeck and associates (1998): developmental assessment, resource linkage, supportive intervention, intervention, advocacy, empowerment, utilization of social learning methods, recognizing the level of prevention and readiness for change, and utilization of the family unit as change agent.

SOCIAL WORK PRACTICE WITH CHILDREN AND FAMILY AND IN HEALTH

One may wonder whether family health as a practice approach is the same as the advanced generalist approach in a family and children or health setting. Although the family health approach employs generalist skills, as discussed, it is not advanced generalist. Therefore, it certainly is not an advanced generalist approach with a focus on family and health.

The family health approach as a practice model for social work embodies professional social work values, an interrelated and integrated set of theories, and associated practice skills. This practice approach may be used with clients in various settings with a clear family well-being orientation.

Table 2.1
Comparison of Generalist, Advanced Generalist, and Family Health Practice

Generalist	Advanced Generalist	Family Health
Assesses at multiple levels	Adds more complex assessment skills	Adds perspectives on health and family to assessment
Problem solving	Problem solving	Problem solving and promotion of holistic well-being
Limited autonomy in practice settings	Independent practice	Independent practice and expertise in family and health interventions
Broker skills as general skill	Broker of more complex situations	Interactional and reflective practitioner as broker of family health practice
Advocacy skills as general skill	Advocacy skills in more complex situations	Advocacy skills on complex health and family issues
Evaluator skills as general skill	Evaluator skills in more complex situations	Evaluator of health and family issues and practice
Basic manager skills awareness	Expectation of managing skills in agency	Expertise in management of service systems serving health and family issues
Social justice view	Social justice view	Social justice view
Basic awareness of family issues	Increased awareness of family issues	Highly developed knowledge on family health issues
Policy analysis as general skill	Policy analysis in more complex situation	Policy analysis and practice in family health context

Social work practice with family and children or in health care settings is defined in terms of the field of practice, target population, or practice settings in which social workers function. Although social workers in these practice settings perform according to the same social work professional values, they may employ relevant but very different social work theories and skills. These theories and skills are not necessarily compatible or structured with an organized orientation as is the case for the family health approach. The orientation of the family health approach to the well-being of the family and its organized theoretical base and practice skills distinguish it from the general practice with children and family and in health and mental health settings.

FUTURE DEVELOPMENT OF FAMILY HEALTH APPROACH

The properties and uniqueness of the family health approach will be better understood as it further evolves. Adopting from Johnson's (1995) framework on social work practice, the following are some guidelines in the future development of the properties of family health approach:

1. As a response to concern, it addresses common human needs. Attention is given to human growth and development, human diversity, related social policy and research issues, and the utilization of ecosystem and social constructivist perspectives.
2. As a developing approach that it will continue to evolve within the professional social work practice context and the social welfare environment.
3. As a creative blending of knowledge, values, and skills that will continue to develop its linkages to other social work theories and approaches. Ongoing inquiries of the appropriateness and adequacy of its technology are necessary and desirable. It should further develop both its descriptive and prescriptive practice skills. The development of the family health approach is guided by social work values and adheres to the social work professional code of ethics.
4. As a social work process that promotes holistic health and well-being through a problem-solving approach, utilizing strength perspectives, empowerment, and the exploration of meaningful realities for the individuals and families as well as the profession.
5. As an intervention into human transactions that focuess on the dynamic of the interplay among individuals, families, and related ecosystems. Important concerns include human diversity, social justice, and at-risk populations. It is a multilevel practice that is informed by current theories and research and guided by professional values and a code of ethics. Most important, it is a goal-oriented intervention approach that aims at achieving the well-being of the family and its members.

REFERENCES

Germain, C. (1983). Technological advances. In A. Rosenblatt & D. Waldfogel (Eds.), *Handbook of clinical social work* (pp. 26–57). San Francisco: Jossey-Bass.

Gibbs, P., Locke, B., & Lohmann, R. (1990). Paradigm for the generalist-advanced generalist continuum. *Journal of Social Work Education, 3*, 232–243.

Johnson, L. C. (1995). *Social work practice: A generalist approach* (5th ed.). Boston: Allyn & Bacon.

Kirst-Ashman, K. K., & Hull, G. H. (1997). *Generalist practice with organizations and communities*. Chicago: Nelson Hall.

Landon, P. S. (1995). Generalist and advanced generalist practice. In R. L. Edwards (Ed.), *Encyclopedia of social work* (19th ed., pp. 1101–1108). Washington, DC: NASW Press.

Pardeck, J. T. (1996). *Social work practice: An ecological approach.* Westport, CT: Auburn House.

Pardeck, J. T., & Yuen, F.K.O. (1997). A family health approach to social work practice. *Family Therapy, 2*(24), 115–128.

Pardeck, J. T., Yuen, F.K.O., Daley, B., & Hawkins, K. (1998). Social work assessment and intervention through family health practice. *Family Therapy, 1*(25), 25–39.

Reynolds, P. (1971). *A primer in theory construction.* Indianapolis: Bobbs-Merrill.

Schatz, M., Jenkins, L., & Sheafor, B. (1990). Milford redefined: A model of initial and advanced generalist social work. *Journal of Social Work Education, 26*(3), 217–231.

School of Social Work, Southwest Missouri State University. (1996). *A working paper on family health.* Springfield, MO: Author.

Wiersma, W. (1969). *Research methods in education.* Philadelphia: J. B. Lippincott.

3

Family Health Social Work Practice: From Theory to Intervention

James G. Daley and Catherine L. Hawkins

This chapter reviews some of the underpinning theories pertinent to family health social work practice, introduces a conceptual framework which incorporates many of the principles of those theories, and integrates that framework into specific interventions that family health social workers provide. The authors describe a case example that illustrates the linkage of conceptual framework to intervention selections. The chapter concludes with a discussion of future directions for theory and intervention development.

AN INCREASING FOCUS ON FAMILIES IN HEALTH CARE DELIVERY

Social work is increasingly emphasizing the importance of the family as a unit of attention, whether trying to ameliorate significant dysfunction or enhance wellness or resilience (Hartman & Laird, 1983; Weick & Saleebey, 1995). Areas of social work intervention include family-centered practice (Cole, 1995; Hartman & Laird, 1983; Kelley, 1996; Laird, 1995; Powell, 1996), family-based services (Pecora, Fraser, Nelson, McCroskey, & Meezan, 1995), family preservation (Denby, Curtis, & Alford, 1998; Faria, 1994; Ronnau & Marlow, 1993; Wells & Biegel,

1991), family practice (Pinderhughes, 1995; Vosler, 1996), family support services (Comer & Fraser, 1998; Lightburn & Kemp, 1994), family strengths approach (Duncan & Brown, 1992; Weick & Saleebey, 1995; Werrbach, 1996), community-centered family services (Sviridoff & Ryan, 1997), family problem solving (Reid, 1985), social work with families (Munson, 1980), and family health social work practice (Pardeck & Yuen, 1997; Pardeck, Yuen, Daley, & Hawkins, 1998; Weick, 1986; Weick & Saleebey, 1995). Space limitations within this chapter prevent a detailed contrast of the models. The main point is that there is extensive attention to how social workers can intervene with families to navigate episodes of illness or facilitate wellness.

Other disciplines have also devoted much effort to family health practice. One intriguing example is the blending of medicine and family therapy, especially the family health and illness cycle model of William J. Doherty and Thomas L. Campbell (Campbell, 1986; McDaniel, Hepworth, & Doherty, 1992, 1997). Concurrently, family nursing is developing increasingly elaborate models for family wellness and health promotion (Bomar, 1996; Feetham, Meister, Bell, & Gilliss, 1993; Friedman, 1992).

Family Health Social Work Practice seeks to glean from this multidisciplinary melting pot of concepts a model that will be useful for enhancing family wellness. It is challenging to converge such diverse theory and model development into a single model of practice. Thus our goal is to be more selective rather than comprehensive in building our model of practice. Our focus is on combining wellness concepts and family intervention strategies to produce a fruitful approach that maximizes family potential. The first step in creating that approach is a clear understanding of the theoretical context.

UNDERPINNING THEORIES OF FAMILY HEALTH SOCIAL WORK PRACTICE

Family Health Social Work Practice merges two large areas of theory and model building: family theories and health/wellness theories. The intent is to blend the interface of the two areas into a new conceptual model, adapt established intervention strategies into that arena of practice, and provide a practice-based modality for social workers to utilize in empowering clients. The goal of family health social work practice is to absorb the best components of a multidisciplinary field of interest and produce a widely applicable framework.

All frameworks must begin with a theoretical basis. But what is a theory?—"a collection of related statements, or propositions that attempt to describe, explain, or predict a particular aspect of experience" (Queralt, 1996, p. 11). In our case, the "experience" is family health. Queralt further asserts that the merit of a theory is directly linked to its parsimony, comprehensiveness, inclusiveness, relevance to practice and everyday life, testability and empirical support, and predictive power. Therefore, the theories gleaned for use with *Family Health Social Work Practice* should be the most robust. One might advocate for another criteria: Measurements should be a rapid assessment form usable for outcome and process assessment (Corcoran, 1997; Stern, 1990). This criteria would certainly enhance the utility by practitioners.

Family Theories

There are dozens of family theories with varying degrees of ability to meet Queralt's (1996) criteria for theory credibility (Gurman & Kniskern, 1981; Janzen & Harris, 1997; Klein & White, 1996; Nichols & Schwartz, 1995). Family theories are becoming increasingly sophisticated. Speculative models based on anecdotal data and practice wisdom are being replaced by models based on solid empirical evidence, clear model components linked to family measurement strategies, and an expectation of multicultural and full-spectrum age consideration (Sawin & Harrigan, 1995).

Most theories still fall short on measurement scales that are directly linked to assessing the constructs of the theory. Most of the established family therapy models have little empirical validation (Sandberg, Johnson, Dermer, Gfeller-Strouts, Seibold, Stringer-Seibold, Hutchings, Andrews, & Miller, 1997), and very few have measurement instruments (especially rapid assessment forms) that assess their basic constructs. More empirically validated models have been demonstrated in models developed to assess family functioning (Sawin & Harrigan, 1995). Some of the best-known models are the Family Competence Model (Hampson, Hulgus, & Beavers, 1991; Lewis, Beavers, Gossett, & Phillips, 1976), the Circumplex Model (Olson, 1991; Olson, Russell, & Sprenkle, 1989), the Family Resiliency Model (formerly called the Double ABCX Model; McCubbin, McCubbin, & Thompson, 1996), and the McMaster Model of Family Functioning (Epstein, Baldwin, & Bishop, 1983; Epstein, Bishop, & Levin, 1978). Each model has clear conceptual themes, a measurement strategy (self-report, observational, or both), operationalization of the themes, and a continuum of healthy or effective functioning. (In this book see chapter 6 by James G. Daley for additional discussion of the concepts, measures, and empirical work on each of the three models.)

In comparing the four models, several issues become apparent. First, the Resiliency Model absorbs the Circumplex Model constructs within its "patterns of functioning" component. Second, whereas the Family Competence Model and the McMaster Model of Family Functioning are family infrastructure concepts, the Resiliency Model focuses more on family adaptation to stress. In other words, two models could be blended together and represent family functioning (McMaster) and family adaptation (Resiliency). Third, a comparison of the three family functioning models indicates the best pick. David Olson's Circumplex Model has some construct validity flaws (Daley, Sowers-Hoag, & Thyer, 1991). Beavers's Self-Report Family Inventory has less confirmatory testing than McMaster's Family Assessment Device (Sawin & Harrigan, 1995; also see table 6.1 in the Daley chapter in this book).

Finally, the Resiliency Model adds a new element to the other models by indicating the process families go through during normative or unanticipated stressors. In sum, the authors advocate that a "best-fit" family assessment model would be a blend of McMaster's structural assessment and Hamilton McCubbin's Resiliency coping factors. As seen later in this chapter, the authors incorporate these elements into the family health impact model.

Wellness/Health Theories

Prevention efforts toward families is not a new idea for social workers (Cyr & Wattenberg, 1957; Geismar, 1969; Rapoport, 1961, 1962; Wittman, 1961). Though often social workers intervene at a family's most devastated moment, the authors always advocate that earliest possible intervention is the most potent approach. A classic public health model is to divide intervention into primary prevention (prior to problem onset), secondary prevention (early in problem development), and tertiary prevention (damage control after the problem is out of control; Leavell & Clark, 1965). These terms have been adapted in the family health promotion literature to family health promotion (primary), family health prevention (secondary), and family symptom removal (tertiary; Loveland-Cherry, 1996; Pender, 1996). Thus a wellness or health focus would center on intervening as close to a family health promotion level as possible.

There are numerous theories about which factors impact on the likelihood of a client (or family) adopting and maintaining a health promotion lifestyle. Table 3.1 outlines 13 health protection or promotion theories, their concepts, whether a formal measure has been developed to assess the components of the theory, and a central reference on the theory. As can be seen from table 3.1, only 3 of the 13 theories focus on the family, and only 3 of the 13 theories (and none of the family health theories) have a formal measure linked to them.

Though a few theories acknowledge environmental influences (often as mediating factors at best), most primarily emphasize individual characteristics (e.g., self-efficacy) as the dominant reasons health promotion occurs. The most complete family health promotion model is Loveland-Cherry's (1996) Family Health Promotion Model. Unfortunately, the model does not have a measure to assess the constructs. However, the theoretical model has significant potential and is incorporated into the Family Health Impact Model.

THE FAMILY HEALTH IMPACT MODEL

Absorbing some of the theoretical perspectives on family functioning and wellness, the authors sought to develop a model that reflected the potent impact the family can have on the health of its members and the community at large. The intent is to visually demonstrate the dual ''ripple pools of change'' that can occur when family health social workers intervene (see figure 3.1). The most effective prevention ripple effect is at the health promotion level. Less significant impact occurs at health protection, and least impact occurs at symptom removal. Concurrently, the authors advocate that societal health promotion can be most significantly effected by family health promotion.

The model also highlights the importance of assessing both family functioning and wellness level. The authors adopt heavily from McMaster's Model, the Resiliency Model, and the Family Health Promotion Model. In addition, they highlight the unique social work value base, generalist skills, and ethical perspective brought to the family intervention. Thus the model incorporates many of the principles of those theories.

Table 3.1
Theories for Understanding Health Protection and Promotion*

THEORY	CONCEPTS	MEASURE**	REFERENCE
Health Belief Model	Threat to health, benefit to act, barriers to act, cues to act, psychosocial variables	None	Janz & Becker, 1984
Protection Motivation Theory	Vulnerable to threat, threat serious, response efficacy, self-efficacy	None	Maddox & Rogers, 1983
Theory of Reasoned Action and Planned Behavior	Intent to act, attitude toward behavior, social norm of behavior, control over behavior	None	Ajzen, 1988
Self-Efficacy Theory	Cumulative self efficacy	None	Bandura, 1986
Theory of Interpersonal Behavior	Intent to act, habit strength, environmental influence, arousal level to act	None	Triandis, 1977
Cognitive Evaluation Theory	Self-determination, intrinsic motivation, extrinsic reward to act, control over act	None	Deci & Ryan, 1985
Interaction Model of Client Health Behavior	Demographics, social influence, past experience with behavior, environment, intrinsic motivation, cognitive appraisal, affective response, affective support, health information, decisional control, technical competencies	Health Self -Determinism Index HSDI for Children	Cox, 1982 Cox, 1985 Cox, Cowell, Marion, & Miller, 1990
Relapse Prevention Theory	Decreased self-efficacy, lapse, abstinence violation effect, relapse	None	Marlatt & Gordon, 1985
Stages of Change Theory	Pre-contemplation, contemplation, action, maintenance	Stages of Change Scale	Prochaska & DiClemente, 1984

Health Promotion Model	Importance of health, control of health, self-efficacy, definition of health, view of health status, benefit of acting, barriers to acting, demographics, biological factors, interpersonal influences, situational factors, behavioral factors, activity-related affect, commitment to act, immediate competing demands and preferences	Health Promoting Lifestyle Profile	Pender, 1996
Family Health and Illness Cycle	5 stages: family health promotion and risk reduction, family vulnerability and disease onset or relapse, family illness appraisal, family acute response, family adaptation to illness or recovery	None	McDaniel, Hepworth & Doherty, 1992
Family Cycle of Health and Illness	8 phases: family health, family vulnerability and symptom experience, sick role and family appraisal, medical contact and diagnosis, illness career and family adjustment, recovery and rehabilitation, chronic adaptation, death and family reorganization	None	Danielson, Hamel-Bissell & Winsted-Fry, 1993
Family Health Promotion Model	Family system patterns, demographics, biological factors, family health socialization patterns, family definition of health, perceived family health status, barriers to act, benefits to act, prior results of acting, family norms on health promotion, intersystem support for acting, situational influences on acting	None	Loveland-Cherry, 1996

*Portions of this table are adapted from a discussion in chapter 2 of Pender (1996).

**This column is specifically asking for a measure that captures the concepts of the model. When the answer is "none," it means there are no measures that capture this model. However, many of the theories/models have had numerous empirical studies done verifying the validity of the model by survey, epidemiological assessment, etc. But the theory or model does not have a measure that could be used by assessor of client.

Figure 3.1
Family Health Impact Model: "Two Ripple Pools of Change"

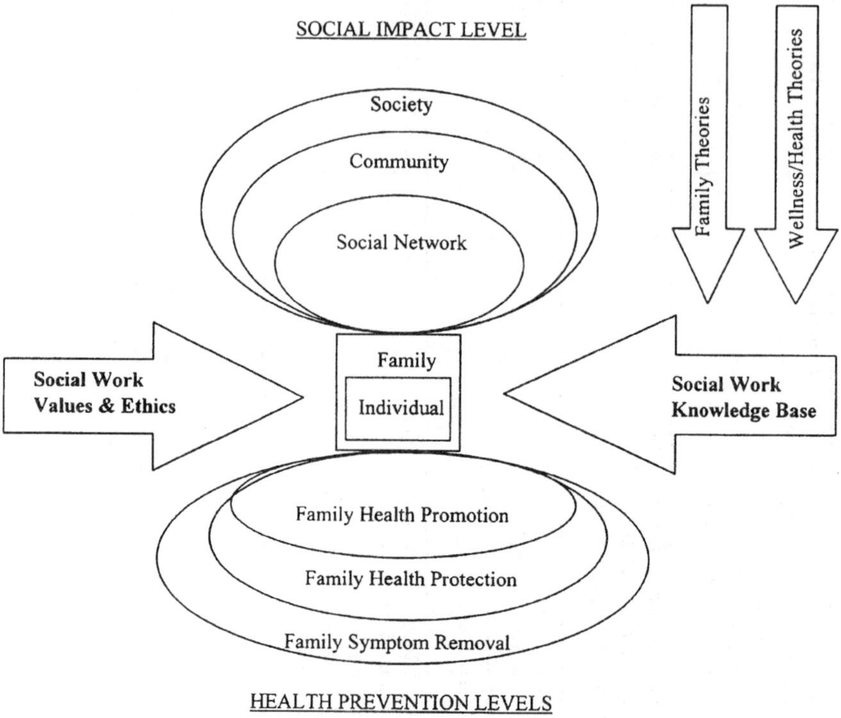

Specific Interventions Linked to Family Health Impact Model

Family health social work practitioners blend two skill components: generalist and family health. Most MSW-level social workers have training in at least a generalist perspective that includes intervention at the individual, family, group, organization, and community level. In essence, the generalist is the jack-of-all-trades who provides the skills needed for the job to get done. Family health social work practitioners utilize that training extensively but also have specialized training in family interviewing, family assessment and intervention, knowledge of medical care systems, and awareness of health/wellness models of family empowerment.

The family health social work practitioner would offer intervention strategies such as:

1. Apply an assessment of the blend of individual, family, and community factors involved in facilitating family wellness.
2. Navigate the intervention process from preparation, assessment, intervention, evaluation of results, and termination. The family health social worker maximizes involvement of the family in each stage of the process and incorporates wellness and family health promotion into the process.
3. Utilize the social context of the agency to help the family system (e.g., knowledge of resource choices, awareness of the agency mission, linking the client family with needed programs, reducing inappropriate barriers).
4. Apply a life-course, trauma-aware, and diversity- and justice-enhancing perspective to the family system.
5. Focus strengths building and wellness parameters to reduce barriers to effective family functioning.
6. Define the central client issues, critique the pertinent scholarly literature, and refine the information to contribute to useful assessment and intervention strategies.
7. Demonstrate the ability to skillfully navigate family interviewing on sensitive issues.
8. Apply practice evaluation technology to confirm that intervention strategies work.
9. Facilitate the family unit's role as multiplier of each member's ability and potential.

But the reality is that family health social work practice is a blend of family health skills, generalist skills, and client-unique issues. Table 3.2 contrasts the three different aspects of any case.

The wild card factor is always what the client system (person, family, community) is seeking and willing to work on. The meshing together of the three components results in what happens in practice. Now let's look at how this model might unfold with a case.

CASE EXAMPLE DEMONSTRATING FAMILY HEALTH SOCIAL WORK PRACTICE

Joe and Mary Smith arrived at 8 P.M. with their three children (8-year-old Annie, 5-year-old Ben, and 6-month-old John) at the Iowa Hotel, a

Table 3.2
Intervention Skills for Family Health Social Work Practice

GENERALIST SKILLS	CLIENT UNIQUE SKILLS	FAMILY HEALTH SKILLS
Resource finder	Diversity issues	Developmental assessment
Client advocate	Specifics of problem	Sensitivity to family issues
Client educator	Readiness for change level	Family assessment skills
Micro/mezzo/macro intervention	Resource needs	Sensitivity to medical care system as context
Administrator	Trauma history	Family intervention skills
Clinical intervention	Family and social linkages	Wellness and prevention focus
Supportive skills	Willingness to accept help	Family empowerment

temporary housing site for the indigent. The police brought them to the hotel from the bus station. The Smiths said they had left Arizona because they had heard that New Haven, a nearby resort town, had lots of jobs—but upon arrival at New Haven they discovered no jobs and nowhere to stay, even for one night. The New Haven Salvation Army recommended that they go to the Iowa Hotel in Springfield.

Joe describes himself as a skilled carpenter. Mary admits to a drinking problem and describes son Ben as "retarded." The case is assigned to Helen Ready, a family health social work practitioner who is working at the Iowa Hotel. She does an initial developmental screening of each of the children and links them with a family physician who volunteers at the hotel. Ready's initial assessment indicates significant language delay and cognitive impairment in Ben and high suspicion of failure to thrive (FTT) in John; she highlights these findings for the physician and coordinates with Department of Family Services (DFS) on the FTT possibility.

Ready begins discussion with the parents on resources available (food stamps, Aid for Families With Dependent Children) but also observes the couple's interaction with each other and the children. Joe seems distant and only perks up when employment issues are raised, while Mary seems to provide the primary nurturing and structure within the family. The practitioner slowly develops a broader understanding through a genogram and ecomap of their family and social supports and determines very limited social connections or bonding with the family of origin.

The social worker begins building on the family's strengths by including them in choices of resources sought, prioritizing which problem to focus on initially. The family decides that Joe's employment, stable housing, and financial help are their top concerns. Helen raises the issue of Mary's drinking problem, but Mary describes having not had a drink for six weeks since she completed a substance abuse treatment program. Helen suggests that a local substance abuse rehabilitation program has an aftercare program that waives the fee for indigent clients. Mary concurs that aftercare sessions would help her.

The family health practitioner follows the family as Joe seeks employment; DFS investigates and provides assistance with the FTT issue (expediting Medicaid coverage, working with the family on feeding problems with John, serving as link with the family physician); Mary gets support with her substance abuse recovery; and Annie and Ben begin school. The family health practitioner encourages improvement in communication skills and slowly gains some credibility with Joe about the usefulness of a more egalitarian parenting style and the value of attachment efforts with John. The practitioner beams as she sees the family move out of the Iowa Hotel into a Housing Authority apartment.

The practitioner has shown a variety of skills consistent with the family health model: a thorough biopsychosocial assessment, resource linkage within an empowerment framework, providing support and confrontation, and advocating for the client when needed. She timed her interventions for the readiness stage of the family for different helping strategies and worked to prevent tertiary problems as much as possible. Finally, she maintained a focus on the family unit as the best resource for change and stability. She uses all of her resources, both internal and external, for the good of her clients.

FUTURE DIRECTIONS FOR THEORY AND INTERVENTION DEVELOPMENT

This chapter has illustrated that much work has been done on theory development on families and wellness, but scant on family health promotion. Further, some theory-linked measures exist, but much more measurement development is needed. The authors have proposed a new model that has yet to be empirically tested and has no direct measure linked to it. These are top priorities for research. The rapidly growing involvement of nursing and medicine in family health promotion indicates a fertile multidisciplinary arena for model development. The impact of environmental (especially macropractice) variables on family wellness is an area of research scarcely touched. In sum, there is a limitless range of research needs in this growing area of practice.

REFERENCES

Ajzen, I. (1988). *Attitudes, personality and behaviors*. Chicago: Dorsey Press.

Bandura, A. (1986). *Social foundations of thought and action: A social cognitive theory*. Englewood Cliffs, NJ: Prentice-Hall.

Bomar, P. J. (Ed.). (1996). *Nurses and family health promotion: Concepts, assessment, and interventions* (2nd ed.). Philadelphia: W. B. Saunders.

Campbell, T. L. (1986). Family's impact on health: A critical review. *Family Systems Medicine, 4*(2–3), 135–323.

Cole, E. S. (1995). Becoming family centered: Child welfare's challenge. *Families in Society, 76*(3), 163–172.

Comer, E. W., & Fraser, M. W. (1998). Evaluation of six family support programs: Are they effective? *Families in Society, 79*(2), 134–148.

Corcoran, K. (1997). Use of rapid assessment instruments as outcomes measures. In E. J. Mullen & J. L. Magnabosco (Eds.), *Outcomes measurement in the human services: Cross-cutting issues and methods* (pp. 137–143). Washington, DC: NASW Press.

Cox, C. (1982). An interaction model of client health behavior: Theoretical prescription for nursing. *Advances in Nursing Sciences, 5*, 41–56.

Cox, C. (1985). The health self-determinism index. *Nursing Research, 34*(3), 177–183.

Cox, C. L., Cowell, J. M., Marion, L. N., & Miller, E. H. (1990). The health self-determinism index for children. *Research in Nursing Health, 13*(4), 237–246.

Cyr, F. E., & Wattenberg, S. H. (1957). Social work in a preventive program of maternal and child health. *Social Work, 2*(3), 32–38.

Daley, J. G., Sowers-Hoag, K. M., & Thyer, B. A. (1991). Construct validity of the Circumplex Model of family functioning. *Journal of Social Service Research, 15*(1–2), 131–147.

Danielson, C. B., Hamel-Bissell, B., & Winsted-Fry, P. (Eds.). (1993). *Families, health and illness: Perspectives on coping and intervention*. St. Louis, MO: Mosby.

Deci, E. L., & Ryan, R. M. (1985). *Intrinsic motivation and self-determination in human behavior*. New York: Plenum Press.

Denby, R. W., Curtis, C. M., & Alford, K. A. (1998). Family preservation services and special populations: The invisible target. *Families in Society, 79*(1), 3–14.

Duncan, S. F., & Brown, G. (1992). RENEW: A program for building remarried family strengths. *Families in Society, 73*(3), 149–158.

Epstein, N. B., Baldwin, L. M., & Bishop, D. S. (1983). The McMaster Family Assessment Device. *Journal of Marital and Family Therapy, 9*(2), 171–180.

Epstein, N. B., Bishop, D. S., & Levin, S. (1978). The McMaster Model of Family Functioning. *Journal of Marriage and Family Counseling, 4*, 19–31.

Faria, G. (1994). Training for family preservation practice with lesbian families. *Families in Society, 75*(7), 416–422.

Feetham, S. L., Meister, S. B., Bell, J. M., & Gilliss, C. L. (Eds.). (1993). *The nursing of families: Theory, research, education, practice*. Newbury Park, CA: Sage.

Friedman, M. M. (1992). *Family nursing: Theory and practice* (3rd ed.). Norwalk, CT: Appleton & Lange.

Geismar, L. L. (1969). *Preventive intervention in social work*. Metuchen, NJ: Scarecrow Press.

Gurman, A. S., & Kniskern, D. P. (1981). *Handbook of family therapy* (Vols. I & II). New York: Brunner/Mazel.

Hampson, R. B., Hulgus, Y. F., & Beavers, W. R. (1991). Comparisons of self-report measures of the Beavers System Model and Olson's Circumplex Model. *Journal of Family Psychology, 4*, 326–340.

Hartman, A., & Laird, J. (1983). *Family-centered social work practice*. New York: Free Press.

Janz, N. K., & Becker, M. H. (1984). The health belief model: A decade later. *Health Education Quarterly, 11*(1), 1–47.

Janzen, C., & Harris, O. (1997). *Family treatment in social work practice* (3rd ed.). Itasca, IL: F. E. Peacock.

Kelley, P. (1996). Family-centered practice with stepfamilies. *Families in Society, 77*(9), 535–544.

Klein, D. M., & White, J. M. (1996). *Family theories: An introduction*. Thousand Oaks, CA: Sage.

Laird, J. (1995). Family-centered practice in the postmodern era. *Families in Society, 76*(3), 150–162.

Leavell, H., & Clark, A. E. (1965). *Preventive medicine for doctors in the community*. New York: McGraw Hill.

Lewis, J. M., Beavers, W. R., Gossett, J. T., & Phillips, V. A. (1976). *No single thread: Psychological health in family systems*. New York: Brunner/Mazel.

Lightburn, A., & Kemp, S. P. (1994). Family support programs: Opportunities for community-based practice. *Families in Society, 75*(1), 16–26.

Loveland-Cherry, C. J. (1996). Family health promotion and health protection. In P. J. Bomar (Ed.), *Nurses and family health promotion* (2nd ed., pp. 22–35). Philadelphia: W. B. Saunders.

Maddox, J. E., & Rogers, R. W. (1983). Protection motivation and self-efficacy: A revised theory of fear appeals and attitude change. *Journal of Experimental and Social Psychology, 19*, 469–479.

Marlatt, G. A., & Gordon, J. R. (1985). *Relapse prevention: Maintenance strategies in the treatment of addictive behaviors*. New York: Guilford Press.

McCubbin, H. I., McCubbin, A. I., & Thompson, M. A. (1996). *Family assessment: Resiliency, coping and adaptation—Inventories for research and practice*. Madison: University of Wisconsin Press.

McDaniel, S. H., Hepworth, J., & Doherty, W. J. (1992). *Medical family therapy: A biopsychosocial approach to families with health problems*. New York: Basic Books.

McDaniel, S. H., Hepworth, J., & Doherty, W. J. (1997). *The shared experience of illness: Stories of patients, families, and their therapists*. New York: Basic Books.

Munson, C. E. (Ed.). (1980). *Social work with families: Theory and practice*. New York: Free Press.

Nichols, M. P., & Schwartz, R. C. (1995). *Family therapy: Concepts and methods* (3rd ed.). Boston: Allyn & Bacon.

Olson, D. (1991). Commentary: Three-Dimensional (3-D) Circumplex Model and revised scoring of FACES II. *Family Process, 30,* 74–79.

Olson, D., Russell, C. S., & Sprenkle, D. H. (1989). *Circumplex Model: Systematic assessment and treatment of families.* Binghamton, NY: Haworth Press.

Pardeck, J. T., & Yuen, F.K.O. (1997). A family health approach to social work practice. *Family Therapy, 24*(2), 115–128.

Pardeck, J. T., Yuen, F.K.O., Daley, J. G., & Hawkins, C. (1998). Social work assessment and intervention through family health practice. *Family Therapy, 25*(1), 25–39.

Pecora, P. J., Fraser, M. W., Nelson, K. E., McCroskey, J., & Meezan, W. (1995). *Evaluating family-based services.* New York: Aldine De Gruyter.

Pender, N. J. (1996). *Health promotion in nursing practice* (3rd ed.). Stamford, CT: Appleton & Lange.

Pinderhughes, E. (1995). Empowering diverse populations: Family practice in the 21st century. *Families in Society, 76*(3), 131–140.

Powell, J. Y. (1996). A schema for family-centered practice. *Families in Society, 77*(7), 446–448.

Prochaska, J. O., & DiClemente, C. C. (1984). *The transtheoretical approach: Crossing traditional boundaries of change.* Homewood, IL: Dow Jones-Irwin.

Queralt, M. (1996). *The social environment and human behavior: A diversity perspective.* Needham Heights, MA: Allyn & Bacon.

Rapoport, L. (1961). The concept of prevention in social work. *Social Work, 6*(1), 3–12.

Rapoport, L. (1962). Working with families in crisis: An exploration in preventive intervention. *Social Work, 7*(3), 4–47.

Reid, W. J. (1985). *Family problem solving.* New York: Columbia University Press.

Ronnau, J. P., & Marlow, C. R. (1993). Family preservation, poverty, and the value of diversity. *Families in Society, 74*(9), 538–544.

Sandberg, J. G., Johnson, L. N., Dermer, S. B., Gfeller-Strouts, L. L., Seibold, J. M., Stringer-Seibold, T. A., Hutchings, J. B., Andrews, R. L., & Miller, R. B. (1997). Demonstrated efficacy of models of marriage and family therapy: An update of Gurman, Kniskern & Pinsof's chart. *American Journal of Family Therapy, 25*(2), 121–137.

Sawin, K. J., & Harrigan, M. P. (1995). *Measures of family functioning for research and practice.* New York: Springer.

Stern, S. B. (1990). Single-system designs in family-centered social work practice. In L. Videka-Sherman & W. J. Reid (Eds.), *Advances in clinical social work research* (pp. 48–53). Washington, DC: NASW Press.

Sviridoff, M., & Ryan, W. (1997). Community-centered family service. *Families in Society, 78*(2), 128–139.

Triandis, H. C. (1977). *Interpersonal behavior theory.* Monterey, CA: Brooks/Cole.

Vosler, N. R. (1996). *New approaches to family practice: Confronting economic stress.* Thousand Oaks, CA: Sage.

Weick, A. (1986). The philosophical context of a health model of social work. *Social Casework, 67*(10), 551–559.

Weick, A., & Saleebey, D. (1995). Supporting family strengths: Orienting policy and practice toward the 21st century. *Families in Society, 76*(3), 141–149.

Wells, K., & Biegel, D. E. (Eds.). (1991). *Family preservation services: Research and evaluation.* Newbury Park, CA: Sage.

Werrbach, G. B. (1996). Family strengths-based intensive child case management. *Families in Society, 77*(4), 216–226.

Wittman, M. (1961). Preventive social work: A goal for practice and education. *Social Work, 6*(1), 19–28.

4

Treating Families Through a Family Health Perspective

Mary Ann Jennings and Gregory J. Skibinski

The previous chapter described family health assessment strategies, which emphasize the strengths and capabilities of families to resolve their own problems. Once those capabilities are identified, the question becomes "How does the family resolve its problems?" The purpose of this chapter is to translate the family health perspective into social work practice principles and strategies that build on the assessment process. To do this the authors begin by (a) briefly revisiting the family health approach to practice and its underlying principles and values and (b) suggesting intervention strategies using a family health perspective. Because wellness is the foundation of the family health perspective, the authors draw heavily upon the strengths perspective and resiliency literature in describing practice principles and strategies. They also extend the principles of wellness and strengths to a family's environment as ecological theory undergirds family health practice described in this chapter.

FAMILY HEALTH

The family health perspective is more detailed than the title implies. Just as problems can beset a family from a number of areas, intervention from the family health perspective is also a strategy that demands more than the application of some theory of family therapy. Family health is a wellness perspective in the broadest sense of the term. It is not just concerned with making families happy and healthy, but also removing obstacles and problems like deficit models, using family strengths to accomplish those goals, and achieving a state of wellness that can prevent future problems. Family health is a perspective that encompasses prevention, correction, and coping strategies for intractable problems and allows the worker to use the strengths of the family and its members to achieve wellness. It is not tied to any one theory or system size but focuses on a family's well-being.

Living in today's society has become increasingly difficult because of the multiple roles people hold in this fast-paced world. The simpler times of a farm economy, ice cream socials at church, representational politics, and single-income families have been replaced by an international economy, politically active religious groups, interest group politics, and two-income families who utilize day care and chauffeur kids to soccer practice. Consequently, families and family members carry more routine responsibilities and may experience more stress than their predecessors.

Indeed, a strong organism is defined as one in robust, sound health, with qualities of solidarity, endurance, and power. This power includes the "inherent capacity of individuals to grow and change and become more" (Weick, 1986, p. 554) and to heal themselves, using internal and external resources. Therefore, optimal functioning relies on positive, helpful transactions with one's environment.

As a player or perhaps a pinball in the larger environment, social, psychological, political, economic, and other sources may affect the family or its members. The problem may have an internal locus such as alcoholism or an external origin (e.g., economic recession). Only the former is readily amenable to traditional family therapy. Problems with external origins may require assistance from other professionals (e.g., physicians), may take long to accomplish (e.g., developing adequate day care in the neighborhood), or simply be intractable (e.g., a terminal illness).

There are many methods of intervention to a person's problems, and some will be more effective than others. What may be the most effective approach, however, is family health—as the family may be a source of strength and support for the therapeutic process. What distinguishes family health from other approaches is its focus on the family and its health. As such, it is a wellness model focused on the most powerful and dependent relationship grouping in society. Family can be defined in many ways, such as a dyad, a large family, or a single person who maintains some affiliation with his or her loved ones. But regardless of society's definition of a family, what is important for the person in need is her or his own definition of family. For example, in most states, homosexual relationships are not legally considered family, yet homosexual couples often define themselves as a family. A family is whatever a client defines in his or her mind as a family. It is a postmodern/social constructionist view and is likely to facilitate change, as the social worker will be consistent with the clients' view of themselves and their social situation.

Health is also broadly defined. Health can be viewed "as a manifestation of the continuous interaction between physical and social processes both internal and external to the individual" and, therefore, "is based on a complex view of causality" (Weick, 1986, p. 554). For the family health practitioner it includes not only physical health but mental, emotional, social, spiritual, and economic well-being. Health has a positive connotation for intervention because it is strength focused. The goal is not necessarily to alleviate some deficit but to establish a state of wellness, making the person, persons, or family the best they can be. It is a self-actualization model for families. It does not imply that intervention must focus only on strengths, especially if a problem under the control of the family or its members can be assuaged. Ignoring such an intervention can aggravate the problem.

Within the context of this book, this view of health is extended to the family unit. The definition of family health offered in this book emphasizes the developmental, interactional, and nonstatic nature of health, which in turn implies its amenability to change and the capacity of family members to learn and grow. The principles and strategies defining family health practice should reflect these benchmarks.

FAMILY HEALTH PRACTICE PRINCIPLES

Because the family health perspective emphasizes the capacities of human beings, the practice principles are drawn from the concepts of the strengths, ecological, resiliency, and empowerment perspectives of human behavior. Although these concepts are considered separately, many of their principles overlap and support those of the others.

Strengths Perspective

The strengths perspective is a holistic approach, one that considers the capacities of individuals, families, and environments. The focus is on strengths and not on pathology or deficits. "Trauma and abuse, illness and struggles may be injurious, but they may also be sources of challenge and opportunity" (Saleebey, 1997, p. 13), a principle that highlights the resilient capacities of individuals and environments to grow, learn, and change.

The strengths perspective offers three practice principles designed to make the best use of those capabilities to allow individuals and communities to heal themselves. First, the social worker–consumer relationship is primary and essential. It is through this relationship that "social and personal resources are activated" (Weick & Chamberlain, 1997, p. 41). Second, aggressive outreach is the preferred mode of intervention. If social workers adopt a holistic approach to knowing and working with their clients, it is imperative they know not only the personal but the social and cultural contexts in which their consumers live. This cannot be accomplished in an office setting that more often highlights the expert and dominant role of the professional (Rapp, 1992).

Third, interventions are based on client self-determination; that is, the client is the director of the helping process. Successful interventions demand dialogue and collaboration between worker and consumer (Saleebey, 1997). This dialogue emphasizes the meaning clients attach to events in their lives; in fact, their meaning "must count for more in the helping process and scientific labels and theories must count for less" (De Jong & Miller, 1995, p. 729). The collaboration includes the cooperative exploration by worker and client to discover these meanings and the strengths clients bring to the helping relationship—the "expert practitioners do not have the last word on what is needed" (De Jong & Miller, 1995, p. 729).

Ecological Perspective

The ecological perspective of considering human behavior complements the strengths perspective, which emphasizes meeting and working with people in their resource-laden environment, and with the systemic view of resilience, which focuses on the interplay of internal and external protective factors. The concept of transactions between human beings and their environment is key in the ecological perspective.

In a complex society, there are many sources of potential problems, and those problems can require elaborate remedies. Even simple remedies may be elusive if the problems or solutions are not under the control of the family. Therefore, the intervention perspective must view the family and its members as interactive environmental participants.

The person-in-the-environment perspective attempts to assess and treat the person in her or his environment. The most immediate environment in which a person interacts is the family—daily and intimately. Family serves as a source of strength, comfort, and at times, problems. The family intermingles with the larger systems of society. The larger environment also plays a role in their lives. Those larger systems can cause problems that are outside the family's and its members' control.

Harold L. Wilensky and Charles N. Lebeaux (1965) believe that the family and the economic institutions can provide for many family needs, but the social welfare institution responds when the other institutions do not. For example, when families cannot properly care for children, the social welfare institution might intervene with day care, foster care, adoption, or financial assistance. Social work and the family health perspective is a part of that social welfare institution. That task can be monumental.

For example, when downsizing leaves employees without a job, there is a direct impact on the family. That family needs to continue to interact with the institutional network and must function in a socially acceptable manner. The family has a right to at least minimal comfort and happiness. But conflicts and roadblocks may appear. Although the family breadwinner has a primary responsibility to her or his family, the unemployed worker cannot steal food for the family's dinner. Society rarely condones crime in the face of hardship. It becomes the social welfare institution's responsibility to eliminate the need for illicit or other unacceptable activity.

"The transactional process suggests that a reciprocal relationship exists between the client and environment. The environment contributes to the client's adjustment, and the client's behaviors create unique responses with the environment; thus, both affect each other" (Pardeck, 1996, p. 4). Therefore, human beings can impact their environments, thus indicating that individuals have abilities and strengths and can rebound from adverse interactions with those environments.

Of primary importance to family health practice is the manner in which the ecological approach moves the focus of assessment and treatment "away from the individual toward the various systems within the client's environment (including the family and community) that comprise the client's larger social ecology" (Pardeck, 1996, p. 4). The ecological, strengths, and resilience perspectives of human behavior require that social workers interact and intervene with clients and their ecosystems.

Resiliency

Resiliency is the ability to recover from trauma and adapt to change. Family health practice relies on the resilient capacities of families to participate in their own healing processes using the concepts of protective and risk factors. Protective factors are those "attributes of individuals and environments, which serve as buffers between a person and stressful situations" while risk factors are those that "if present, increase the likelihood of a person developing an emotional or behavioral problem at some point" (Hawley & DeHaan, 1996, p. 288).

Protective factors are summarized into individual, familial, and contextual/environmental elements. Individual factors include characteristics that elicit positive attention from primary caretakers, for example, an easy, good-natured, and cuddly temperament; an above-average intelligence; a more internal locus of control; effective problem-solving and coping skills; an achievement orientation; the capacity to construct productive meanings for events in their world that enhances their understanding of the events; and positive feelings of self-regard and self-efficacy (Barnard, 1994; Brooks, 1994; Herrenkohl, Herrenkohl, & Egolf, 1994; Luthar & Zigler, 1991; Masten, Best, & Garmezy, 1990; Robinson & Fields, 1983; Werner, 1994).

Familial elements that promote resilience include parents who are competent, loving, and patient and who set rules in the home, parental caring for a child during and after major stresses, and a good relationship between a child and at least one parental figure (Luthar & Zigler, 1991; Masten et al., 1990). Environmental protective elements include networks of informal relationships (e.g., friends, ministers, and in some cases, teachers); positive school relationships; church memberships and faith in a higher power; and connections with institutions that foster ties to the larger community (Herrenkohl et al., 1994; Luthar & Zigler, 1991; Masten et al., 1990). Social workers' efforts are directed at enhancing internal and external protective factors to reduce those that prove to be a risk to clients.

The task of family health practice is to apply these factors to the family unit because while the "relationship between families and individual resilience is well established, the notion of family units being resilient has only recently surfaced in the literature'' (Hawley & DeHaan, 1996, p. 288).

An ecological, developmental perspective of resilience is also consistent with a health-oriented approach to practice that emphasizes internal and external sources of healing. Froma Walsh (1996) comments that to ''understand and encourage psychosocial resilience and protective mechanisms, we must attend to the interplay between what occurs within families and what occurs in the political, economic, social, and racial climates in which individuals perish or thrive'' (p. 266). A developmental perspective demands that families have a ''variety of coping strategies to meet different challenges as they emerge'' (Walsh, p. 267).

Empowerment

In the definition of empowerment by Lisa Kaplan and Judith L. Girard (1994, p. 40), it is evident that as a practice principle, it complements those of the strengths, ecological, and resilience perspectives: ''Empowerment encompasses a way of thinking about families. It's a conviction that families deserve respect, have strengths, *can* make changes in their lives, and are resilient, and it means helping families gain *access* to their power, not giving them power. The worker must believe in the family and communicate that she knows they are capable of getting their needs met and handling their own difficulties.'' According to Kaplan and Girard, the concepts underlying an empowerment approach to family-based services include a pragmatic, hands-on approach designed to treat each family individually; creativity and flexibility on the part of the social worker; and the use of multidimensional interventions, which highlights the necessity to work with clients and their environments.

Summary of Family Health Practice Principles

The strengths, ecological, resiliency, and empowerment perspectives of human behavior are interrelated and complement each other, often using the same terminology in their definitions and concepts. The four approaches all contend that people can learn, grow, and change; that people have the ability to participate actively in and direct the helping process; and that social workers must focus on internal and external processes affecting human behavior and the transactions between individuals and their environments. The emphasis is on capabilities, not just deficits, for it is with strengths and abilities that problems are resolved.

These practice principles require that social workers assume particular roles in their interactions with consumers such as collaborator, advocate, facilitator, ally, broker, and mediator, roles that place consumers in the director's chair and social workers in the assistant's position.

FAMILY HEALTH INTERVENTION STRATEGIES

From the descriptions of family health practice above, it follows that intervention strategies in this model should empower families by enhancing their strengths and resiliency and reflect the ecological perspective of human behavior as well as the essential qualities of social work practice. These are the standards to which the strategies described below will be held. To give an overview of the form family health treatment might take, the authors present four examples of intervention. First, they examine examples of basic social work skills for their applicability to a family health practice model. Second, the authors discuss the applicability of generalist social work practice, in which intervention occurs at multiple levels as needed, to a family health practice model. Third, they consider a solution-focused approach to treatment, and finally, they present aspects of resilient family processes developed by James M. Patterson (1991).

Basic Social Work Practice Skills

To consider the relevance of basic social work skills for family health practice, two particular skills, partializing and reforming, are examined. The discussion of these two skills is designed to promote a critical appraisal of the extent to which other common practice skills empower clients and promote their strengths and resilience.

According to Lawrence Shulman (1992), partializing is essentially a problem-managing skill. The only way to tackle complex problems is to break them down into their component parts and address those parts one at a time. The way to move past the feelings of being immobilized is to begin by taking one small step, working on one part of the problem. Helping a family partialize its problems expresses the social worker's belief that the members can resolve those problems; the underlying premise is that the family has strengths and that those capacities can be marshaled to meet their needs. By breaking overwhelming problems into manageable pieces, the worker helps clients gain access to their own power. Partializing also moves the focus of the intervention away from ''blaming the victim'' by ''focusing on the work, rather than on the client'' (Shulman, 1992, p. 143).

Furthermore, in research conducted by Shulman, partializing was one of many skills that ''contributed to the development of the trust element in the working relationship'' (1992, p. 142). Not only is the client–social worker relationship considered the medium through which helping and change occurs, but positive relationships with persons outside the immediate family are considered a protective factor that reduces stress in the family.

Barry Cournoyer defines reframing as the words and actions a social worker takes when ''introducing clients to a new way of looking at some aspect of themselves, the problem, or the situation. . . . Reframing is applicable when the fixed attitude constitutes a fundamental part of the problem for work'' (1996, p. 337). As with partializing, this skill is premised on the belief that clients can learn and adopt new ways of looking at themselves and their problems and situations. Helping clients assume a different, more workable perspective frees up their internal power to meet their needs, for example, by changing a negative view of themselves into a positive one.

One form of reframing described by Cournoyer (1996), situationalizing meaning, reflects the ecological perspective of human behavior. When situationalizing the meaning of a problem or situation with a client, the social worker suggests that the client's feelings or behaviors may be ''viewed as a result of external, societal, systemic, situational, or other factors beyond the client's individual control or responsibility'' (p. 339).

This discussion of these two skills reveals questions a practitioner should ask when applying any intervention strategy in a family health model. Does the strategy reflect a belief on the worker's part that family members can learn, grow, and change? Does the manner in which the worker applies the skills (e.g., with respect and empathy) reflect this belief? Does the intervention enhance factors that protect the family from stress and promote coping? Does treatment consider and impact factors outside the family that are influencing its members' behaviors and attitudes? Finally, is any skill used by the worker designed to release the power within the family and its circumstances?

A ''yes'' answer to these questions is contingent upon the application of the essential social work qualities to the interventions used. To promote family health, practice skills must reflect empathy, warmth, and respect, because without these basic characteristics, mutuality and collaboration are impossible.

Generalist Social Work Practice

The best source of intervention for a family in need is the family health perspective. The family is a source of strength and personal resources that can and must be mustered for maximum effectiveness. Ideally, the social worker should intervene at the family level, alleviating the problem in the most parsimonious method. However, a problem can arise with the source of the difficulty. What can the social worker do if the roadblock is out of the direct control of the family, such as a plant closing?

A two-prong approach is necessary. If at all possible, the social worker should eliminate the source of the problem. In complex networks of problems, however, that may be time-consuming. In the interim, the social worker should use the strength of the family to help members cope with the situation and change the avenues of institutional interaction when necessary to eliminate the dependence on the source of the problem. For example, in the case of the unemployed worker, the social worker might first try to get the employee's job back or arrange for a transfer to the new plant if that is what the worker would prefer. Simultaneously, the social worker might enlist the help of a psychiatrist for antidepressant drugs, a psychologist for therapy, or refer the employee to a job counseling service while simultaneously supporting and maintaining the integrity of the family unit so that the situation does not spiral out of control, creating other repercussions.

According to Jerome Frank (1982), all clients are demoralized and distressed. It is a function of intrapsychic conflicts with a subsequent loss of self-esteem, a distorted perception of others, and deficient coping skills. Each mutually reinforces the other, leading to a downward spiral and increased demoralization. Intervention, therefore, must break the downward spiral with support, encouragement, and morale building. The source of that strength must be the family, with assistance of the social worker. A generalist social worker finds ways to release the power of both families and the environment to improve their circumstances.

Solution-focused Treatment

Solution-focused treatment is based on the premise that people come to treatment wanting to change their situation and that "no matter how awful and how complex the situation, a small change in one person's behavior can lead to profound and far-reaching differences in the behavior of all persons involved" (De Shazer, Berg, Lipchik, Nunnally,

Molnar, Gingerich, & Weiner-Davis, 1986, p. 209). The emphasis of solution-focused interviewing is on well-formed, concrete goals and exceptions, which are "those occasions in the client's life when the client's problem could have occurred but did not" (De Jong & Miller, 1995, p. 731).

According to Peter De Jong & Scott D. Miller (1995), well-formed goals have several characteristics. Well-formed goals are ones that are important to the family; they belong to the family and are expressed in the family's language. Goals are small and accomplishable; they are concrete, specific, and behavioral. Goals in solution-focused treatment seek the presence rather than the absence of behaviors and are realistic within the context of the client's life.

Such goal setting with consumers reflects family health practice principles and essential social work qualities in several ways. Formulating goals that are important to the family gives preeminence to the family's meaning of events in their lives and demands mutuality and collaboration between social worker and family members. Goals developed by and with families indicate the worker's belief that families want to and can resolve their problems. Goals that belong to families enhance their motivation, which empowers them to achieve their objectives.

Goals that are expressed in the family's language and are specific reflect the concreteness appreciated by clients (Maluccio, 1979). Objectives that are realistic within the context of the family's life demand that workers know and understand the transactions that occur between the family and its environment and intervene with that environment.

Goals that depict the presence rather than the absence of behavior are positive in nature, reflect the strengths people possess, and demonstrate the emphasis on exceptions mentioned earlier. As described by De Jong and Miller, workers using a solution-focused approach to treatment concentrate on "the who, what, when, and where of exception times instead of the who, what, when, and where of problems. The consequence is a growing awareness in both workers and clients of the clients' strengths relative to their goals, rather than the clients' deficiencies relative to their problems" (1995, p. 731). Once families become aware of their strengths, they can be empowered to "mobilize them to create solutions tailor-made for their lives."

Resilient Family Processes

Through a review of the literature on families and disabilities, Patterson (1991) has identified nine traits of resilient family processes:

1. Balancing the illness with other family needs.
2. Maintaining clear family boundaries.
3. Developing communication competence.
4. Attributing positive meanings to the situation.
5. Maintaining family flexibility.
6. Maintaining a commitment to the family as a unit.
7. Engaging in active coping efforts.
8. Maintaining social integration.
9. Developing collaborative relationships with professionals.

These factors serve to protect families from developing behavioral and/or emotional difficulties that would impair their functioning. Therefore, it is important that social workers find ways to help families develop and maintain these characteristics.

An examination of a few of these characteristics reveals their congruity with a family health practice model. First, families who adapt best to a child's disability "use coping strategies to define the situation in a way that makes their circumstances more manageable and they find meaning in what they are experiencing" (Patterson, 1991, p. 495). Helping families reframe their problems and situations so that they are more comprehensible and controllable empowers families to free up their energies to cope more effectively with the difficulties they face.

Second, developing collaborative relationships with professionals demonstrates direct application of the strengths perspective to work with families experiencing stress. A positive working relationship also establishes a positive connection between the family and an institution in their community, a protective factor identified in the resiliency literature. In addition, a collaborative relationship demands that the family and social worker assume codirectorships of the helping process. Therefore, family members are empowered to discover, use, and develop their own strengths and resources to contribute to their healing.

Third, "resilient families are effective, efficient, problem-solving units. They do not passively resign themselves to their circumstances or let someone else manage their child's needs" (Patterson, 1991, p. 496). Again, the strengths perspective is evident in this trait of resilient families. Families are active directors of and participants in their healing processes. This characteristic is premised on the belief that families are capable of resolving their problems and meeting their needs. It is through a productive relationship with a professional that these capabilities are released and utilized.

Finally, maintaining social integration reflects both the ecological and resilience perspectives of human behavior. "Social support is one of the most powerful buffers of high levels of chronic stress for all families" (Patterson, 1991, p. 496). Helping families establish and maintain their systems of social support requires the social worker to consider the family's connections and transactions with its environment. The environment becomes the focus of the worker's attention as she/he works with the family to discover and develop supportive networks.

As with the family health practice strategies introduced earlier, the processes indicative of resilient families are predicated on the essential social work qualities. Collaborative relationships between families and professionals underscore the other traits of resiliency and demand the presence of critical professional qualities such as respect, empathy, concreteness, and genuineness.

Summary of Family Health Practice Intervention Strategies

Basic social work skills such as partializing and reframing, the generalist practice model, solution-focused treatment, and resilient family processes are examples of intervention strategies that reflect and support family health practice. These strategies require workers to establish collaborative relationships with families that allow families to eliminate problems and discover and use their own strengths and abilities. Social workers help families through that discovery process, which may include looking beyond the immediate household to the environment to find needed resources. In all their interactions with families and their environments, social workers strive to fortify those elements which protect and nurture families and diminish those factors that put families at risk for behavioral and emotional problems.

REFERENCES

Barnard, C. P. (1994). Resiliency: A shift in our perception? *American Journal of Family Therapy, 22*, 135–144.

Brooks, R. B. (1994). Children at risk: Fostering resilience and hope. *American Journal of Orthopsychiatry, 64*, 545–553.

Cournoyer, B. (1996). *The social work skills workbook* (2nd ed.). Pacific Grove, CA: Brooks/Cole.

De Jong, P., & Miller, S. D. (1995). How to interview for client strengths. *Social Work, 40*, 729–736.

De Shazer, S., Berg, I. K., Lipchik, E., Nunnally, E., Molnar, A., Gingerich, W., & Weiner-Davis, M. (1986). Brief therapy: Focused solution development. *Family Process, Inc., 25*, 207–221.

Frank, J. (1982). Therapeutic components shared by all psychotherapies. In J. H. Harvey & M. M. Parks (Eds.), *The master lecture series, vol. 1, psychotherapy research and behavior change* (pp. 5–37). Washington, DC: American Psychological Association.

Hawley, D. R., & DeHaan, L. (1996). Toward a definition of family resilience: Integrating life-span and family perspectives. *Family Process, Inc., 35*, 283–298.

Herrenkohl, E. C., Herrenkohl, R. C., & Egolf, B. (1994). Resilient early school-age children from maltreating homes: Outcomes in late adolescence. *American Journal of Orthopsychiatry, 64*, 301–309.

Kaplan, L., & Girard, J. L. (1994). *Strengthening high-risk families: A handbook for practitioners*. New York: Lexington Books.

Luthar, S. S., & Zigler, E. (1991). Vulnerability and competence: A review of research on resilience in childhood. *American Journal of Orthopsychiatry, 61*, 6–22.

Maluccio, A. N. (1979). *Learning from clients: Interpersonal helping as viewed by clients and social workers*. New York: Free Press.

Masten, A. S., Best, K. M., & Garmezy, N. (1990). Resilience and development: Contributions from the study of children who overcome adversity. *Development and Psychopathology, 2*, 425–444.

Pardeck, J. T. (1996). *Social work practice: An ecological approach*. Westport, CT: Auburn House.

Patterson, J. M. (1991). Family resilience to the challenge of a child's disability. *Pediatric Annals, 20*, 491–499.

Rapp, C. A. (1992). The strengths perspective of case management with persons suffering from severe mental illness. In D. Saleebey (Ed.), *The strengths perspective in social work practice* (pp. 45–58). New York: Longman.

Robinson, B. E., & Fields, N. H. (1983). Casework with invulnerable children. *Social Work, 28*, 63–65.

Saleebey, D. (1997). Introduction: Power in the people. In D. Saleebey (Ed.), *The strengths perspective in social work practice* (2nd ed., pp. 3–19). New York: Longman.

Shulman, L. (1992). *The skills of helping individuals, families and groups* (3rd ed.). Itasca, IL: F. E. Peacock.

Walsh, F. (1996). The concept of family resilience: Crisis and challenge. *Family Process, Inc., 35*, 261–281.

Weick, A. (1986). The philosophical context of a health model of social work. *Social Casework: The Journal of Contemporary Social Work, 67*, 551–559.

Weick, A., & Chamberlain, R. (1997). Putting problems in their place: Further explorations in the strengths perspective. In D. Saleebey (Ed.), *The strengths perspective in social work practice* (2nd ed., pp. 39–48). New York: Longman.

Werner, E. E. (1994). Overcoming the odds. *Developmental and Behavioral Pediatrics, 15*, 131–136.

Wilensky, H. L., & Lebeaux, C. N. (1965). *Industrial society and social welfare*. New York: Free Press.

5

A Statistical Analysis of Family Health

Dee K. Vernberg

The idea that statistical methods provide a rational means for revealing valid knowledge underlies why governments have used scientific evidence to justify certain decisions and policies regarding health and social welfare (Marcorini, 1988; Rosen, 1955). For similar reasons, clinicians increasingly have come to rely on statistical knowledge to define normative behavior or to evaluate therapeutic and preventive practices. Consequently, statistics are often viewed as a lens through which facts of life and society can be viewed and understood (Starr, 1987). This widely held perspective is illustrated in remarks once made by John F. Kennedy:

> I know that statistics and the details of the economy may sometimes seem dry, but the economy and economic statistics are really a story of all of us as a country and these statistics tell whether we are going forward or standing still or going backward. They tell us whether an unemployed man can get a job or whether a man who has a job can get an increase in salary or own a home or whether he can retire in security or send his children to college. (cited in Scott, 1967, p. 67)

In the same way, statistics of health tell a story about such things as how and when people die, whether children are receiving immunizations, or how many people are unable to work because of functional limitations. Housing statistics, on the other hand, might be used to describe the proportion of families with children that live in crowded and/or inadequate conditions. Statistics, then, are used to paint a picture of groups of people and how the lives of these people change over time. Many decision makers who use these statistics realize that behind every statistic there is a person. They might, for example, acknowledge that people in a democratic society are free to make individual decisions. But users of statistics also presume that culture influences the range of options available to an individual. Thus, statistics are viewed as providing some insights into the lives of people.

Historically, social statistics have provided an important voice for understanding societal institutions such as the family. For example, prevailing notions of what is normative for families, how family structures have changed over time, or how these changes have affected family health are ideas that have emerged from statistical findings. Statistics also define what appear to be risk factors for family problems. Because the family is regarded as a major societal institution, family health often is considered a factor when social problems are studied (Coontz, 1989; McCarthy, 1992). In fact, this view that the family and society interact has shaped statistical analyses of family health so that measures of family often incorporate measures of societal health, and population-based health measures frequently include aspects of family health. Therefore, the statistical analysis of family health can be approached from many different angles, with various types of data, and to answer different types of questions.

This chapter focuses on the analysis of family health from the perspective of official statistics. Other types of statistical analyses that deal with the evaluation or cost benefits of particular treatments or programs aimed at families or children, or that examine different models of risk assessment in clinical populations, do not receive sustained attention. Instead, the emphasis of this discussion centers on how the statistics that governments produce, finance, or routinely incorporate into their decisions (Starr, 1987) shape how family health is understood. In order to accomplish this goal, the chapter investigates questions that pertain to three areas of study:

1. *The sociology of statistics.* Why do official agencies keep statistics? How does the process of collecting statistics shape the way health and family health are viewed?

2. *Statistics as a means of analysis.* What types of information do official statistics provide about the family and family health? What are common indicators of family health, and what indicators are incomplete or lacking?
3. *An epistemological analysis of statistics.* What epistemological assumptions do researchers make when they calculate or interpret statistics? What presuppositions do social scientists and statisticians make regarding knowledge acquisition and the role of the individual? How do these epistemological assumptions help or hinder the development of strategies for enhancing family health?

THE SOCIOLOGY OF OFFICIAL STATISTICS

Statistics are not collected in a social vacuum. For example, how statistical systems collect and analyze data or how findings are interpreted and disseminated raise certain types of questions regarding the meaning of this information and knowledge. Because statistical findings have a potential influence on how social phenomena such as family health are understood, the author considers the origins of statistical systems and describes statistics as a form of scientific discourse. This investigation includes topics such as how statistical systems are justified in democratic societies and a description of the social process of statistical production.

Statistical Systems

The use of statistical analyses to understand health and social problems had its origins in the scientific revolution that occurred in England during the seventeenth century (Montgomery, 1996; Starr, 1987). During this time, the natural philosophers of the Royal Society developed a quantitative technique, political arithmetic, that consisted of observations of population, education, diseases, and revenue. These early scientists asserted that the analysis of these numeric data would reveal objective knowledge that could be used to rationalize affairs of government (Emery, 1993). The implicit or explicit assumption in these arguments was that statistical findings would be used for the public good.

Modern statistical systems in England and the United States were developed on the premise that statistical information could be used to generate value-free knowledge on which fair and sound decisions could be based. For example, in the United States, the statistical system of the census was developed to make decisions regarding representation in the House of Representatives and the Electoral College (Starr, 1987). Statistical findings from vital statistics, on the other hand, were initially sought so that governments and businesses could develop a sound actuarial basis for developing annuities, life insurance, and friendly-society sick benefits (Emery, 1993).

Economic and legal concerns clearly shaped the development of many statistical systems, but these same systems also were strongly influenced by the public health movement. For example, knowledge of mortality patterns was used to empirically justify sanitary reforms in the nineteenth century. Governments, then as now, were interested in ways to improve health and well-being in order to reduce government spending on relief (Emery, 1993).

During the twentieth century, democratic governments increasingly have looked to official statistical systems to provide information to justify public policies in areas such as public health, education, or labor. Consequently, an enormous government knowledge industry has emerged to assess risk and well-being in society (Emery, 1993). The purpose of these systems is to produce certified knowledge that is specific enough to describe group characteristics without posing any risk to individuals. These numbers represent the states' assessment of society, the act of naming groups of people, defining social institutions, and identifying social problems.

There are many potential applications if public data are collected and analyzed, but the production of this knowledge is tempered by general public distrust of governmental activity. Because of the public's suspicion of government, statistical systems in democratic countries and the data they collect must be justified (Starr, 1987). Moreover, the programs that collect statistics operate under strict rules about such things as what data can be collected, what data are public information, how some data may be used, and how findings will be reported. At the same time, public support of statistical systems is garnered by making certain types of data or statistical findings available and accessible. Therefore, a delicate tension exists between the government and the public regarding the collection of official statistics.

In part, public support for official statistics can be attributed to the presumption that data are collected by impersonal, objective bureaucracies and to a trust that adequate safeguards are in place to protect an individual's privacy (Starr, 1987). Because of this expectation, particular care is taken to report data in a way that cannot identify individuals personally. Instead, data are analyzed at the group level. Statistical findings, in turn, serve to define group identity and are used to construct perceptions about how significant various groups are in society. This information also serves to substantiate a particular social order by reporting population-based standards or norms (Starr, 1987).

Production of Official Statistics

A variety of official sources provide data related to family health. Some of the most common data bases include the U.S. Census, death certificates, birth certificates, marriage licenses, divorce records, and these surveys: Consumer Expenditure, National Health Interview, American Housing, National Crime Victimization, National Household Education, and Income and Program Participation. Sometimes administrative data sets such as those collected by social service agencies, insurance companies, or private organizations like the Hospital Association may be used to generate official statistics. These sources of data are used when official sources of data are unavailable to describe an illness or measure the amount and extent of health care utilization in a community.

Regardless of the source, organizational goals define the purpose of data collection, shape the type of data that are collected, influence measurement issues such as operational definitions, and frame the questions that are analyzed and the interpretation of the findings. In other words, the collection of data is a social process directly affected by decisions regarding what type of variables will be collected, how these variables will be operationally defined, who will collect the data, how the data will be computerized and analyzed, and what findings will be distributed. These methodological decisions ultimately define the standardized notions of health and social phenomena. Often referred to as social indicators or measures of well-being, these official definitions influence how issues might be framed, and statistics provide a rational approach for making decisions regarding where prevention programs should be targeted or what groups are labeled at risk.

This social process of statistical production very often is obfuscated, because the decision-making process of producing statistics is rarely discussed (Collier & Toomey, 1997). Furthermore, many of the metaphors used to describe statistical production serve to reinforce the idea that statistics are accurate and powerful by incorporating the imagery of war and technology (Montgomery, 1996). For example, when some types of public health statistical data bases are called surveillance systems, these data are often referred to as a source of social and economic intelligence. Organic and technological metaphors further reinforce the notion that statistics are mirrors or senses through which society can be understood and managed. "A surveillance system is to public health as eyes and ears are to individual people. A more accurate analogy is that of radar—signals going out and coming back—the quintessential elements of a surveillance system" (Hopkins, 1992, p. 87).

Regardless of whether a data source is considered to be a surveillance system, frequently metaphors of war and technology are used when describing these data sets. These images serve to elevate statistical findings to the status of social facts. Thus the language that is used to describe statistical production serves to strengthen the belief that statistics are objective conclusions about phenomena (Montgomery, 1996). Because statistics are viewed as certified knowledge, the validity of findings often is not questioned. By accepting official statistics as knowledge, the public and many professionals tend to embrace these findings in spite of a deep-seated suspicion of governmental activities (Starr, 1987).

STATISTICS AS A MEANS OF ANALYSIS

When statistics are used as a means of analysis, family health usually is described in terms of factors that place families at risk for adverse outcomes or indicators that predict the need for services. The statistical findings of family health, however, may vary among studies, because different dimensions of health may be measured or different living arrangements may be defined as a family. For example, the U.S. Bureau of the Census (Census Bureau, 1996) defines a family as a group of two or more people (one of whom is the householder) living together, who are related by birth, marriage, or adoption.

It is important to note that this definition of the family does not require children to be present. In fact, statistical findings from the Census Bureau (1996) suggested that in 1995, 51% of families had no children under 18 years old at home. However, for some analyses, family is defined as households with children. The focus of these official statistics is on children, youth, and their families. Individuals living alone or with nonrelatives such as boarders or roommates are rarely considered in family health analyses. These living arrangements are referred to as a nonfamily household by the Census Bureau. According to 1995 data, 30% of the U.S. population resided in nonfamily households (Census Bureau, 1996).

Like the concept of family, health may be measured in various ways by official agencies. For example, traditional measures of family health include outcome measures such as infant mortality rates, childhood cause-specific mortality rates (death rates due to firearms, suicide, or cancer), teen birth rates, proportion of low birth weight infants, or use of preventive health care services such as prenatal care. More recently, health surveys have been used to measure morbidity and health behaviors.

Measures of morbidity from health surveys might include estimates of conditions such as depression or activity limitations due to poor physical or mental health. Health behavior measures quantify the prevalence of risk factors such as cigarette smoking, alcohol abuse, illicit drug use, or compliance with recommended preventive measures such as childhood immunizations or screenings (e.g., Pap smear). Other common measures of well-being reported by statistical agencies that relate to family health may include official assessments of economic security, juvenile crime victimization rates, academic achievement, or school completion rates (Federal Interagency Forum on Child and Family Statistics [Federal Interagency Forum], 1997).

Characteristics of the American Family

Most statistical findings describing the American family over the last few decades suggest that there have been substantial changes in the structure of the family. For example, from 1970 to 1996 the number of American children living with two parents dropped from 85% to 68%. Some of this increase in single-parent families can be attributed to the rise in births to unmarried mothers (from 5% in 1960 to 32% in 1995). However, almost two thirds (65%) of children in single-parent households live with a parent who has been formerly married. This increase in single-parent families translates into a substantial number of children: 18.9 million or 27% of all children under the age of 18 in 1995 (Census Bureau, 1997b; Federal Interagency Forum, 1997).

While most (86%) single parents are mothers, statistics between 1970 and 1995 indicated that the number of female and male single parents had risen. For example, from 1970 to 1995 the number of female-headed family groups with children rose from 3.4 million to 9.8 million, and the number of men living with children without a spouse rose from 0.4 million to 1.7 million (Census Bureau, 1994, 1996, 1997b; Federal Interagency Forum, 1997).

A substantial number of children (four million) live in the homes of their grandparents. According to 1995 data, more than one third (37%) of these children lived with their grandparents without their parents, 52% lived with one parent in their grandparents' home, and 11% of these children lived with both of their parents in a grandparents' home (Census Bureau, 1997b).

More than 500,000 children reside in foster care because they cannot remain safely in their own home. Many of these children return to their homes, but more than 100,000 children cannot return to their homes because of safety concerns. These children remain in foster care until they can be placed permanently with an adoptive family. Many of the children living in foster homes who are eligible for adoption are considered to have special needs because they are older; members of a minority or sibling groups; or physically, mentally, or emotionally disabled (Administration for Children and Families, 1998).

Findings Related to Family Health and Well-being

Considerable attention is given to family structure with regard to family health because very often the stability of the home and the number of parents living with a child are related to the quality and amount of human and economic resources available to the child. Children living with one parent, particularly their mother, are more likely to live in poverty. Poverty, in turn, has been shown to be associated with increased health and social risks, such as poor physical and mental health, difficulties in school, exposure to violence, and teenage pregnancy (Census Bureau, 1995, 1997a; Federal Interagency Forum, 1997).

Because so many single parents and their children experience economic disadvantages, official agencies have begun to monitor factors such as prevalence of child support judgments and compliance with these rulings. Official data for 1991 regarding child support payments suggested that about half of custodial mothers (56%) and custodial fathers (41%) had awards for child support. Of these parents, approximately 76% of custodial mothers and 63% of custodial fathers received some or all of their child support. Not surprisingly, single parents who received some or all of their child support payments had higher incomes than single parents who did not receive child support payments (either because the noncustodial parent did not pay or because the custodial parent was not awarded a payment).

Extra income, however, may not be the only child support benefit. Some custodial parents and their children may receive health insurance as part of their child support. In fact, approximately, 41% of the single parents who are awarded child support payments have health insurance included as a benefit. However, almost a third (31%) of these parents do not receive this benefit from the noncustodial parent. With regard to compliance with child support judgments, statistics suggest that noncustodial parents are more likely to pay if they have regular contact with their children. For example, 79.3% of noncustodial parents with visitation and/or joint custody paid child support in 1991, compared to 55.8% of noncustodial parents who did not have visitation or joint custody of the children (Census Bureau, 1995).

Most families depend on secure parental employment and adequate pay for economic security. Not only does employment assist families in avoiding the risks associated with economic deprivation (Roberts, 1997), but jobs are also the means by which most families obtain private health insurance. Official statistics suggest that private health plans provide coverage for 66.3% of children under 18 years old. The Medicaid program provides health care coverage for an additional 21.8% of children. However, many working parents do not have health insurance benefits as part of their jobs. Because many of these parents cannot afford private health insurance, 14.8% (10.6 million) of children under 18 years old do not have access to medical care afforded by this benefit (Census Bureau, 1997c).

The benefits of secure family employment are not directly measured by official statistics, but data from other types of studies suggest that economic security is related to physical and psychological well-being in children, cognitive competence, and stronger family functioning. Presumably, the protective effect of secure family employment is due to decreased stress and other negative effects that are experienced when parents are underemployed or unemployed (Census Bureau, 1997c; Federal Interagency Forum, 1997; Sameroff, 1996).

Although employment outside the home appears to be a protective factor for family health, many families cite work as a source of stress. During the past two to three decades, the proportion of women in the workforce has risen. This trend is especially evident among women with infants and preschool-age children. For example, between 1950 and 1987 the number of women with children under 6 years old working outside the home rose from 11.9% to 56.8%. Moreover, many mothers today return to work shortly after giving birth (Zigler & Stevenson, 1993).

The large number of working mothers translates into a large number of children who must be cared for while the mother works. For example, in 1991, there were 10 million preschoolers who had working mothers. Of these children, approximately two million were cared for in an organized day care such as a nursery school, four million were cared for in their own homes, and three million were cared for in another home (Census Bureau, 1994, 1995). While research has shown that maternal employment does not necessarily have negative effects on children, many working families report severe stress in trying to balance family life and work (Zigler & Stevenson, 1993). Stress, in turn, can have adverse effects on health status and family functioning (Taylor, Repetti, & Seeman, 1997).

These examples of official statistical findings are not intended to represent a comprehensive account of what is known about family health from data collected from governmental agencies. Instead, this description is intended to give the reader a feel for the kinds of information that may be obtained from official statistics. Official agencies collect an enormous amount of data, but significant gaps exist in these data bases when one attempts to study family health. For example, official statistics cannot describe the quality of day-care experiences or aspects of family social environment such as quality of parenting, conflict in the home, or parents' mental health, even though these factors may influence child and adolescent health (Taylor et al., 1997).

Furthermore, the confidentiality or anonymity of many data sets often precludes the comprehensive examination of multiple risk factors that may have a significant impact on child, adolescent, parental, or adult health factors (Sameroff, 1996). Because the unit of analysis for most official statistical analyses is an individual, health or well-being for the entire family is not easily assessed with these data. Some health surveys, such as the National Health Interview, however, allow some aspects of family health to be studied. For example, Sally K. Gallagher and David Mechanic (1996) used the mental health supplement of the National Health Interview Survey to study health outcomes of those living with someone with mental illness. These researchers found that family members living with relatives with mental illness reported poorer physical health and used more medical services than people who did not live in households with members who had mental illness.

While these and other statistical findings are supposed to provide insight into problems so that solutions can be developed, recently some scholars have criticized some statistical analysts for focusing almost exclusively on statistical techniques and having little or no concern for the subject matter. As Mervlyn Susser (1989) warned, this approach tends to create findings that are flat rather than rounded—caricatures rather than portraits. In other words, the passive objectivity of statistical analyses may limit social understanding and hinder problem solving. The epistemological investigation that follows will explore reasons why statistical approaches to family health cannot adequately capture the social context of this topic.

EPISTEMOLOGICAL ANALYSIS OF STATISTICS

On one level statistics can be thought of as tools for analyzing data. On another level, statistics might be conceived of as evidence for describing social phenomena or for arguing that a particular conclusion is valid. Because statistics serve to support what is believed to be knowledge, the author approaches the epistemological analysis of family health statistics in terms of how statistical knowledge is acquired. This discussion focuses on the assumptions underlying scientific methods and statistics and the role of the human mind and rationality in these procedures. The intent of this discussion is twofold: (a) to examine some of the arguments advanced by science to assert that statistical findings represent truth and (b) to address some of the limitations of positivistic social science in understanding family health from a family systems perspective.

Assumptions Underlying Science and Statistics

When statistical findings are presented as facts, researchers are appealing to a belief in universal natural law even if the results are reported as probabilistic statements (Strahler, 1992). This notion involves two beliefs: (a) that the universe or society functions in an orderly and predictable way and (b) that scientific method and empirical study are the most valid ways to discover the natural laws that explain orderly or predictable behavior, that is, cause (Collier & Toomey, 1997).

The assumptions underlying the methods used to produce official statistics can be equated with those inherent in the epistemological theory of realism. This theory states that the world can be understood objectively through observations and calculations (Dreyfus & Dreyfus, 1986; Susser, 1979). Several ideas underlie realism: (a) the natural world is the preferred reality, and (b) scientific methods of observation are the only legitimate means of attaining knowledge.

Positivism as it is employed in the statistical analyses of family health presumes an empirical view of knowledge. This position states that knowledge resides in an objective, material world (Bunge, 1981; Susser, 1979). Thus, what can be observed is real, and what cannot be observed is unimportant or superfluous (Manicas, 1987). By approaching the acquisition of knowledge in this way, emphasis is placed on the method of careful observation and description. This scientific approach allows for findings to be replicated, which in turn provides evidence for arguing that findings are valid (Collier & Toomey, 1997). Therefore, the data used to analyze family health consist of observable variables such as personal attributes (i.e., age, gender, marital status), material possessions or assets (i.e., income, home ownership, poverty level), benefits or services (government assistance, health care utilization), geographical space (residence), or clock/calendar time.

Within the theory of realism, arguments of reliability and validity rest on presuppositions that the world out there is independent of the scientist or the observer. Therefore, officials who produce official statistics attempt to register this reality as accurately as they can. In order to accomplish this goal, methodological procedures demand detached and impartial observation so that biases inherent in subjective perception can be eliminated (Mulkay, 1979). This approach requires the adoption of a dualistic theory of the mind. Dualism presumes that while knowledge might be conceived of as ideas, facts are derived from objective, sense experience (Nicholson, 1939). The purpose of the mind is to act as a blank slate and to register reality as it really is. This process, sometimes referred to as the copy theory of knowledge, demands that researchers purge themselves of emotion and other subjective influences (Murphy, 1989).

The role of reason in scientific methods is to assure that knowledge is not contaminated with personal inclinations, values, or subjectivity. As explained by Phillip Slater, "the essence of what we call rational thought is leaving out things. The most important thing it leaves out is the thinker—his or her unique location in the universe, with its associated urges, feelings and motives. Rational thought pretends it does not reside in a person that it is cosmic, unemotional, and unmotivated" (cited in Nathanson, 1985, p. 104).

This emphasis on objectivity presumes that scientific thinking is rational. Calculations or statistical analyses are another dimension of rationality because these systematic procedures are presumed to enhance thinking so that objective truths can be defended in rational argument (Dreyfus & Dreyfus, 1986). As René Descartes argued, the methodological rules of reason allow scientists not only to acquire knowledge but also to assert that findings represent truth as opposed to opinion or mere speculation. The method of reason always starts with the simple and moves step by step to the complex. Therefore, statistical analyses represent a rational method for explaining phenomena by breaking up a complex event into simpler elements (Haugeland, 1985; Nicholson, 1939).

Those who assert that scientists are open-minded, disinterested, and skeptical present statistical findings as though these facts were derived from pure experience, that is, independent of theories and values. Scientists often invoke reason to argue that their decisions are unbiased (Collier & Toomey, 1997) and to assert that statistical findings should be used as an impartial arbiter of scientific controversy (Pera, 1994). Thus, the prestige of official statistics arises from the belief that these statistics symbolize calculative rationality rather than shallow talk (Dreyfus & Dreyfus, 1986; Pera, 1994). Likewise, statistical analyses of family health are presumed to be objective facts rather than ideas that may be influenced by politics or values.

The epistemological assumptions of objectivity, universality, and determinism underlying statistical analyses create findings that are detached and descriptive, an onlooker's analytical understanding of collective [relationships] (Toulmin, 1976). In other words, the dualistic philosophy that maintains the body is separate from the mind elevates the environment and social forces and diminishes the importance of personal contact and human interaction. The result is that statistical analyses transform social and cultural factors such as family history, age, gender, occupation, and community into impersonal social facts or indicators. This mechanistic approach of studying reality by reducing the whole to its individual parts discounts the experiential aspects of living and leads to a conception of people as passive entities (Cooter, 1982).

By assuming individuals merely respond or react to external forces, statistical analyses treat the family as thinglike. This maneuver allows only the physical aspects of the family to be considered. The result is that findings tend to frame family health problems as existing in a social vacuum. Consequently causal explanations are more likely to be physical attributes rather than social processes (Eyler, 1979). Policymakers consider family health statistics as outcome measures, and they use these facts for planning and evaluation purposes. The next section illustrates how statistical findings influence the development of many family health programs and policies.

INFLUENCE OF STATISTICAL FINDINGS ON FAMILY PROGRAMS AND POLICIES

From a public health point of view, the purpose of public health knowledge is to provide a rational basis for public policy and treatment decisions. Frequently this knowledge is presumed to be objective evidence that is acquired solely from scientific studies. This assumption, however, does not accurately reflect how most program policies are actually made. In fact, statistical evidence does not always persuade audiences such as legislators to act (Reardon, 1991; Reinard, 1988). Instead, public policies are much more likely to be enacted if statistical evidence, which defines a hazard or program effectiveness, is coupled with community support (Nelkin, 1989; Sandman, Miller, Johnson, & Weinstein, 1993). Thus, policy decisions are influenced by quantitative and qualitative information.

Public health agencies that are involved in policy development are responsible for developing a broad-based understanding of community needs and resources (Institute of Medicine, 1988). However, most official health needs are documented in terms of quantitative objectives or goals. Because many state programs specifically address health objectives contained in the document entitled *Healthy People 2000*, this section describes the focus of this government publication and of *Healthy People 2010*, the document that soon will replace *Healthy People 2000*.

The purpose of the *Healthy People* documents is to quantitatively define health indicators for the country. These statistical measures also are used to monitor national changes in health status. Three goals are addressed in *Healthy People 2000*: (a) to increase the span of healthy life for Americans, (b) to reduce health disparities among Americans, and (c) to achieve access to preventive services for all Americans. *Healthy People 2010* focuses on the same goals, but also includes the goal of access to quality health care (*Healthy People 2000 Fact Sheet*, 1998). Printed in the fall of 1998, *Healthy People 2010* attempts to incorporate the notion that health improvement begins at home with what we do individually, in families, and in communities to promote mental and physical health (*Developing Objectives for Healthy People 2010, Part 2, [Developing Objectives*], 1998). Therefore, specific risk-reduction objectives are likely to address how to strengthen community prevention. Also, more attention is likely to be paid to functional limitations as a health indicator, the needs of people with disabilities, and on issues related to public health infrastructure.

Although the *Healthy People* documents are not considered to be mandates for the nation, this publication has influenced some national legislation. For example, the Maternal and Child Health Program and Title V of the Social Security Act are now required by law to report progress that states are making toward accomplishing the objectives specified in the Maternal and Child Health targets found in *Healthy People 2000.* Likewise, since 1992, the Preventive Health and Health Services Block Grant program has required state grant-funded programs to address objectives found in *Healthy People 2000.* States that accept these grant monies must have a plan that specifies health focus areas or priorities and at-risk populations to be served by state health prevention and promotion programs. These states must also evaluate how health status is affected by these interventions or services (*Healthy People 2000 Fact Sheet*, 1998).

Many of these state plans, usually entitled Healthy [State] 2000, contain a subset of objectives found in *Healthy People 2000.* Clinicians who are involved in writing grants for preventive services may wish to obtain a copy of their state plan from their State Department of Health. Table 5.1 shows the proposed structure of *Healthy People 2010.* The overall vision for this document is derived from the World Health Organization's Health for All strategy (*Developing Objectives*, 1998). Many of the proposed focus areas could have a direct impact on family health status.

CONCLUSION

In summary, official statistics are influential because they are used to define many public health problems, and this knowledge is used to justify where state and federal prevention resources will be allocated. Long considered to be objective measures of truth, official assessments of risk do not always translate into statements of safety. Because the assumptions underlying statistical methodology do not allow the interpretive aspects of these problems to be measured, official statistics can only contribute to risk management strategies by providing information about high-risk groups or high-risk geographical areas.

This type of knowledge may be used to support decisions for why an intervention is targeted to a specific group or location, but risk assessment information usually is not very useful in developing a specific approach or intervention. For insight into risk management, practitioners must look to other theories and types of research. The importance of official statistics to practice is that funding opportunities for innovative

Table 5.1
Proposed Structure for Healthy People, 2010

Goals	Focus Areas
Increase years of healthy life	Mental, physical impairment & disability; chronic diseases (heart disease, cancer, stroke, lung disease, diabetes)
Promote healthy behaviors*	Physical activity; nutrition, sexual health (HIV and STD), unintentional injuries, tobacco, substance abuse
Protect health*	Food and drug safety, environmental health, occupational health, infectious diseases
Assure access to quality health care*	Health services (clinical preventive, emergency medicine, long-term care), mental health, oral health, family planning, maternal infant & child health
Strengthening community prevention*	Public health infrastructure (research, surveillance), education & community programs, violent/abusive behavior
Eliminate health disparities	Special populations (low-income, minorities, age, people with disabilities)

*Enabling Goal.

Note: Adapted from *Developing Objectives for Healthy People*, 2010, http://www.health.gov/healthypeople/Guide/guide2.htm, 3/13/98.

programs are often linked to official objectives. Thus, successful community practitioners must be aware of official health objectives and must be able to develop persuasive arguments that show how social service interventions address these risk and service objectives.

REFERENCES

The Administration for Children and Families. (1998, January). *Home page.* http://www.acf.dhhs.gov/programs/opa/facts/major.htm.

Bunge, M. (1981). *Scientific materialism.* Dordrecht: Reidel.

Collier, J. H., & Toomey, D. M. (1997). Scientific and technical communication in context. In J. H. Collier & D. M. Toomey (Eds.), *Scientific and technical communication: Theory, practice, and policy* (pp. 3–37). Thousand Oaks, CA: Sage.

Coontz, S. (1989). *America's families: Rhetoric and reality.* Olympia, WA: Evergreen State College.

Cooter, R. (1982). Anticontagionism and history's medical record. In P. Wright & A. Treacher (Eds.), *The problem with medical knowledge: Examining the social construction of medicine* (pp. 58–71). Edinburgh: Edinburgh University Press.

Developing objectives for healthy people 2010, part 2. (1998, March 13). http://www.health.gov/healthypeople/Guide/guide2.htm.

Dreyfus, H. L., & Dreyfus, S. E. (1986). *Mind over machine: The power of human intuition and expertise in the era of the computer.* New York: Free Press.

Emery, G. N. (1993). *Facts of life: The social construction of vital statistics, Ontario, 1869–1952.* Montreal: McGill-Queens University Press.

Eyler, J. E. (1979). *Victorian social medicine: The ideas and methods of William Farr.* Baltimore, MD: Johns Hopkins University Press.

Federal Interagency Forum on Child and Family Statistics. (1997). *America's children: Key national indicators of well-being.* Available from National Maternal and Child Health Bureau Clearinghouse or http://www.cdc.gov/nchswww/nchshome.htm.

Gallagher, S. K., & Mechanic, D. (1996). Living with the mentally ill: Effects on the health and functioning of other household members. *Social Science and Medicine, 42,* 1691–1701.

Haugeland, J. (1985). *Artificial intelligence: The very idea.* Cambridge, MA: MIT Press.

Healthy people 2000 fact sheet. (1998, March 14). http://odphp.osophs.dhhs.gov/pubs/hp2000/hp2kfct1.htm.

Hopkins, D. R. (1992). Public health surveillance: Where are we? Where are we going? *Morbidity and Mortality Weekly Report, 41*(Supplement), 5–9.

Institute of Medicine, Committee for the Study of the Future of Public Health. (1988). *The future of public health.* Washington, DC: National Academy Press.

Manicas, P. T. (1987). *A history and philosophy of the social sciences.* New York: Basil Blackwell.

Marcorini, E. (Ed.). (1988). *The history of science and technology: A narrative chronology* (Prehistory 1900). New York: Facts on File.

McCarthy, A. R. (1992). The American family. In L. Kaplan (Ed.), *Education and the family* (pp. 13–26). Needham Heights, MA: Allyn and Bacon.

Montgomery, S. (1996). *The scientific voice.* New York: Guilford.

Mulkay, M. (1979). *Science and the sociology of knowledge*. London: George Allen & Unwin.

Murphy, J. W. (1989). *Postmodern social analysis and criticism*. New York: Praeger.

Nathanson, S. (1985). *The ideal of rationality*. Atlantic Highlands, NJ: Humanities Press International.

Nelkin, D. (1989). Communicating technological risk: The social construction of risk perception. *Annual Review of Public Health, 10*, 95–113.

Nicholson, J. A. (1939). *An introductory course in philosophy*. New York: Macmillan.

Pera, M. (1994). *The discourses of science*. Chicago: University of Chicago Press.

Reardon, K. K. (1991). *Persuasion in practice*. Newbury Park, CA: Sage.

Reinard, J. C. (1988). The empirical study of the persuasive effects of evidence: The status after fifty years of research. *Human Communications Research, 15*, 3–59.

Roberts, E. M. (1997). Neighborhood social environments and the distribution of low birthweight in Chicago. *American Journal of Public Health, 87*, 597–603.

Rosen, G. (1955). Problems in the application of statistical analysis to questions of health: 1700–1880. *Journal of the History of Medicine, 29*, 27–49.

Sameroff, A. (1996, August). *Democratic and Republican models of development: Paradigms or perspectives*. Presidential address presented at the 104th annual meeting of the American Psychological Association, Toronto, Ontario, Canada.

Sandman, P. M., Miller, P. M., Johnson, B. B., & Weinstein, N. D. (1993). Agency communication, community outrage, and perception of risk: Three simulation experiments. *Risk Analysis, 13*, 585–598.

Scott, A. H. (1967). *Census U.S.A.: Fact finding for the American people, 1790–1970*. New York: Seabury Press.

Starr, P. (1987). The sociology of official statistics. In W. Alonzo & P. Starr (Eds.), *The politics of numbers* (pp. 7–57). New York: Russell Sage.

Strahler, A. N. (1992). *Understanding science: An introduction to concepts and issues*. Buffalo, NY: Prometheus Books.

Susser, M. (1979). *Causal thinking in the health sciences: Concepts and strategies of epidemiology*. New York: Oxford University Press.

Susser, M. (1989). Epidemiology today: A thought-tormented world. *International Journal of Epidemiology, 18*, 481–488.

Taylor, S. E., Repetti, R. L., & Seeman, T. (1997). Health psychology: What is an unhealthy environment and how does it get under the skin? *Annual Review of Psychology, 48*, 411–437.

Toulmin, S. (1976). On the nature of physicians' understanding. *Journal of Medicine and Philosophy, 1*, 32–50.

U.S. Bureau of the Census. (1994). *How we're changing: Demographic state of the nation: 1995* (Current population reports, series P23–188). Washington, DC: U.S. Government Printing Office.

U.S. Bureau of the Census. (1995). *Population profile of the United States, 1995* (Current population reports, series P23–189). Washington, DC: U.S. Government Printing Office.

U.S. Bureau of the Census. (1996). *Household and family characteristics: March, 1995* (Current population reports, series P20–488). Washington, DC: U.S. Government Printing Office.

U.S. Bureau of the Census. (1997a). *America's children at risk* (Census Brief 97–2). Washington, DC: Author.

U.S. Bureau of the Census. (1997b). *Children with single parents: How they fare* (Census Brief 97–1). Washington, DC: Author.

U.S. Bureau of the Census. (1997c). *Health insurance coverage: 1996* (Current population reports, series P60–199). Washington, DC: U.S. Government Printing Office.

Zigler, E. F., & Stevenson, M. F. (1993). *Children in a changing world: Development and social issues* (3rd ed.). Pacific Grove, CA: Brooks/Cole.

6

Clinical Instruments for Assessing Family Health

James G. Daley

The purpose of this chapter is to provide an overview of available measurement strategies for capturing family health as a construct and how those strategies can be applied in a clinical setting. After a brief discussion of the increasing need for formal assessment tools in today's practice arena, the chapter emphasizes some of the theoretical models for family functioning and for the health/wellness perspective. The author outlines measures available to assess family functioning and health/wellness measures. He then illustrates the blending of the theoretical models and measures to produce a useful measurement approach in clinical settings. The chapter concludes with a discussion of the next steps in research on family health social work practice.

THE RAPIDLY GROWING DEMAND FOR FORMAL MEASUREMENT IN CLINICAL PRACTICE

Social work practice has long debated the importance of measuring what we do in clinical intervention with clients (Bloom, Fischer, & Orme, 1995; Hudson, 1982; Nurius & Hudson, 1993). Opponents fiercely resist any measurement touting the complexity of practice, the inadequacy of measurement tools, and the reductionistic process of any formal assessment. Advocates fiercely fight for accountability of practice and demonstration of effectiveness and point to the growing choices of valid and reliable measures to use in practice.

Additional fuel to the argument has been added as the managed care tsunami has emphasized outcome measurement as a key component of effective practice (Brown, 1994; Daley & Bostock, 1998; Kunnes, 1992). Managed care programs are rapidly sifting out practitioners who do not use some form of measurement of practice and embracing clinicians who can systematically produce outcome data (Frankel, 1992; Mizrahi, 1993). With an increasing proportion of social service and mental health services being absorbed by the managed care framework (Bennett, 1993; Dorwart, 1990), social work practitioners are being faced with having to incorporate formal measurement into their practice methods.

As clinicians have sought formal measurement tools to use in practice, they have discovered a wide range of individual (Fischer & Corcoran, 1994; Hudson, 1992) and family (McCubbin, Thompson, & McCubbin, 1996; Sawin & Harrigan, 1995) assessment tools which could be used in clinical practice settings. For example, Joel Fischer and Kevin Corcoran's (1994) two-volume set on *Measures for Clinical Practice* outlines over 262 different self-report measures, Hudson's (1992) *WALMYR Assessment Scales Scoring Manual* gives 22 scales, Sawin and Harrigan's (1995) *Measures of Family Functioning for Research and Practice* describes 17 measures. In addition, dozens of new scales are emerging in the literature every year.

In short, the clinician seeking formal assessment tools can find a wide range in today's literature. These tools enhance the clinician's ability to prosper in a managed care environment and provide on-target assistance to the client system.

KEY CONSIDERATIONS IN ASSESSING FAMILY HEALTH

Models of Family Functioning

Before deciding on a family measure, a clinician should (if at all possible) decide what theoretical framework the measure reflects. The utility of a theoretical framework is the ability to conceptualize where you are going with the client. The measure gives you a point on a map; the map is the theory. Three models are described to illustrate: the McMaster Model of Family Functioning (Miller, Epstein, Bishop, & Keitner, 1985), the Family Resiliency Model (McCubbin et al., 1996), and the Circumplex Model (Olson, 1991).

According to the McMaster Model of Family Functioning, family health is derived from the family's ability to problem-solve, directly communicate, have clear affective and instrumental roles defined and implemented, effectively maintain affective involvement and responsiveness, and have a cooperative but effective mechanism to control behavior within the family when needed. The McMaster model includes a 60-item self-report measure, a clinical rating scale that the clinician could fill out, a structured interview schedule, and a treatment approach (problem-centered systems therapy of the family) directly linked to theoretical constructs. Further, the focus of the model is on how the family functions in all settings, not just when a problem arises. The theoretical constructs fit into a holistic view of families (like gears in a watch).

The Family Resiliency Model of Family Functioning is based on the assumption that all families have stressors. What makes the difference between family health and distress is how they navigate those stressors. The family's ability to maintain balance and harmony hinges on a combination of the family's established patterns of functioning, resources, problem-solving skills, and how they perceive the stressor. Of course, a large enough pileup of stressors can overwhelm any family. The advocates of this model focus on ways to stabilize and strengthen the family system by targeting the weak links in the combination of factors mentioned above. If the family strengthens the weak link, they empower themselves to enhance their family health. McCubbin's program at the University of Wisconsin has an elaborate combination of self-report measures linked to different aspects of the family resiliency theoretical model. Though they have no specific treatment framework or clinician rating format, the McCubbin group have worked hard to make the scales short, easy to use in clinical settings, and clear in what they measure.

The Circumplex Model of Family Functioning advocates that two dimensions, family cohesion and adaptability, are the center of how well the family functions. Specifically, the expectation is that a balanced, mid-range position on each dimension is the healthiest location. In other words, too much or too little family cohesion is problematic. The target for the family is a mid-range level of cohesion.

Though there have been some challenges to the theoretical validity of the model (Daley, Sowers-Hoag, & Thyer, 1990, 1991; Eckblad, 1991; Green, Harris, Forte, & Robinson, 1991), the Olson advocates are working to make a health-focused model that has theory linked with measurement and a focus on enhancing families. Olson's group at the University of Minnesota created the Circumplex Model of family functioning more than 20 years ago and are on the fourth version of their short (20-item) self-report measure (FACES-IV). They also have a clinician rating form that allows an observational scoring, not just self-report completion of the form. There is purposefully not a therapy approach with the Circumplex Model, as the advocates expect it to apply (as an outcome measure) for whatever approach is selected.

Each of the family functioning models has basic tenets, measures linked to those tenets, and some concept of what makes a family healthy. But these models are not the only choices for family functioning measurement. Table 6.1 demonstrates the range of measurement choices, the constructs measured, and some of the advantages of the measure (size of the scale, languages that the scale is available in).

The reader should notice that the measures range from being specifically problem focused (e.g., family discord, prejudice) to being optimum health focused (e.g., communication, financial well-being, optimism). The savvy clinician can pick the measures that link with the health and empowerment focus of the family being evaluated.

Models of Wellness Functioning

Models for understanding how we define health or wellness differ quite dramatically. Three models will be contrasted: the health promotion model (Lusk, Kerr, & Baer, 1995; Pender, 1984), the Wellness Institute's growth model (Palombi, 1992; Travis, 1981), and the psychological well-being model (Ryff & Keyes, 1995). Readers wanting to pursue further models are directed to an excellent qualitative research meta-analysis and model (Jensen & Allen, 1994), an intriguing psychological wellness model (Cowen, 1994), and a cancer-focused wellness model (Zimpfer, 1992).

Nola J. Pender's health promotion model (originating with Smith, 1981) has four dimensions: clinical health (relief from disease), role performance health (fulfilling role requirements), adaptive health (adapting to environment), and eudaimonistic health (fulfilled & self-actualized). The model has developed an instrument, Laffrey's Health Conception Scale, which captures these constructs.

The Wellness Institute developed a growth model concurrently with a self-report measure (Wellness Inventory) that has 12 dimensions: self-responsibility and love, breathing, sensing, eating, moving, feeling,

Table 6.1
Available Measures for Use in Family Functioning Measurement

MEASURE	SOURCE	LANGUAGE	SIZE	CONSTRUCT(S)
Family Assessment Device[a, e]	[Sawin & Harrigan, 1995] [Miller et.al., in press]	1,2,3,4,5,6,7	60	Problem-solving, communication, roles, affective involvement, affective responsiveness, behavior control
Index of Family Relations[b,d]	[Hudson, 1992]	1	25	Family discord
Index of Marital Satisfaction[b,d]	[Hudson, 1992]	1	25	Marital discord
Index of Sexual Satisfaction[b,d]	[Hudson, 1992]	1	25	Sexual discord
Index of Parental Attitudes[b,d]	[Hudson, 1992]	1	25	Parent conflict with child
Child's Attitude toward Mother[b,d]	[Hudson, 1992]	1	25	Child conflict with mother
Child's Attitude toward Father[b,d]	[Hudson, 1992]	1	25	Child conflict with father
Index of Brother Relations[b,d]	[Hudson, 1992]	1	25	Sibling conflict
Index of Sister Relations[b,d]	[Hudson, 1992]	1	25	Sibling conflict
Family Adaptability & Cohesion Scale (FACES II-IV)[b,f]	[Olson, et.al., 1985]	1	20	Family cohesion, family adaptability
Family Environment Scale[a,e]	[Sawin & Harrigan, 1995]; [Moos, 1990]	1,2,4,8,9, 10, 11	90	Cohesion, conflict, control, moral- religious

Table 6.1 (continued)

Feetham Family Functioning[a,f]	**[Sawin & Harrigan, 1995]; [Feetham, 1991]**	**1, 2, 13, 14**	**25**	**Relationship between family and individual, relationship between family and subsystems, relationship between family and broader community**
Family Assessment Measure[b,e]	**[Sawin & Harrigan, 1995] [Skinner, 1987]**	**1**	**134**	**Role performance,communication, affective expression, affective involvement, control, values & norms**
Family Dynamics Measure[a,e]	**[Sawin & Harrigan, 1995] [Lasky et.al., 1985]**	**1, 15, 16, 17,18, 19, 20**	**62**	**Individuation, flexibility, roles, communication, stability, mutuality**
Family Inventory of Life Events and Changes (FILE)[a,g]	**[McCubbin et.al., 1996]**	**1, 6,8,10**	**71**	**Intrafamily strains, marital strains, pregnancy and child bearing strains, financing and business strains, work-family transitions & strains, illness and family "care" strains, losses, transitions "in and out", family legal violations**
Adolescent Family Inventory of Life Events and Changes[a,g]	**[McCubbin et.al., 1996]**	**1,6**	**50**	**Transitions, sexuality, losses, responsibilities and strains, substance use, legal conflict**
Young Adult Family Inventory of Life Events and Changes[a,g]	**[McCubbin et.al., 1996]**	**1**	**70**	**Family stress index (family disruption, family losses and conflicts, health disabilities, financial worries, breaking away- independence, extended family struggles, family transitions, college stress index (pressures,**

				transportation & isolation, limited friendship support and isolation, college advisors and counselors difficulties, study hassles, conflicts between personal values and expectations)
Family Pressures Scale-Ethnic[b,h]	**[McCubbin et.al., 1996]**	**1**	**64**	**Prejudice & family pressures focused on Native Americans**
Family Hardiness Index (FHI)[a,f]	**[McCubbin et.al., 1996]**	**1,6**	**20**	**Commitment, challenge, control**
Family Inventory of Resources Management[a,g]	**[McCubbin et.al, 1996]**	**1**	**69**	**Family strengths (esteem, communication , mastery, health), extended family social support, financial well-being**
Family Time & Routines Index[a,f]	**[McCubbin et.al., 1996]**	**1**	**32**	**Child routines, couple togetherness, meals together, parent-child togetherness, family togetherness, relative's connection, family chores, family management**
Family Traditions Scale[a,f]	**[McCubbin et.al, 1996]**	**1**	**20**	**Holiday traditions, change traditions, religious occasions, family special events**
Family Celebrations Index[a,f]	**[McCubbin, et.al., 1996]**	**1**	**9**	**Scope & depth of celebrations**
Social Support Index (SSI)[a,f]	**[McCubbin et.al., 1996]**	**1**	**17**	**Degree of community support for family**
Coping Health Inventory for Parents (CHIP)[a,g]	**[McCubbin et.al., 1996]**	**1,6**	**45**	**Pattern I (integration, cooperation, optimism), pattern II (support, esteem, stability), pattern III (medical communication & consultation)**

Table 6.1 (continued)

Family Crisis Oriented Personal Evaluation Scales (FCOPES)[a,g]	[McCubbin et.al., 1996]	1,2,6,8	30	Acquiring social support, reframing, seeking spiritual support, mobilizing family acquire and accept help, passive appraisal
Family Coping Index[a,g]	[McCubbin et.al., 1996]	1	24	Seeking professional and spiritual guidance,seeking family and neighbor support, affirming the family's confidence
Adolescent-Coping Orientation Problem Experiences[a,g]	[McCubbin et.al., 1996]	1,2,6, 12,17	54	Ventilating feelings, seeking diversions, developing self- for reliance and optimism, developing social support, solving family problems, avoiding problems, seeking spiritual support, investing in close friends, seeking professional support, engaging in demanding activity, being humorous, relaxing
Family Coping Inventory[a,g]	[McCubbin et.al., 1996]	1	70	Spousal coping with permanent, extended or short-term separation from family: maintaining family integrity, developing interpersonal relationships & social support, managing psychological tension & strain, acceptance of lifestyle & optimism, developing self reliance & self esteem, balanced coping strategy
Family problem Solving Communication[a,g]	[McCubbin et.al., 1996]	1,6	10	Incendiary communication, affirming communication

Dual Employed Coping Scales[a,f]	**[McCubbin et.al., 1996]**	**1**	**58**	**Maintaining family system, procurement of support, modifying roles and standards, maintaining perspective and reducing tension**
Family Coping Coherence Index[a,f]	**[McCubbin et.al., 1996]**	**1**	**4**	**Use of family coherence to cope**
Family Schema - Ethnic[a,g]	**[McCubbin et.al., 1996]**	**1**	**39**	**Degree of which a schema (world view including ethnicity) is part of family identity**
Family Attachment and Changeability Index 8[a,g]	**[McCubbin et.al., 1996]**	**1,6**	**16**	**Attachment, changeability (has different cut-off scores for African American and Caucasian clients)**
Family Member Well Being Index[a,g]	**[McCubbin et.al., 1996]**	**1**	**8**	**Overall view of emotional, social, interactional and physical well-being**
Family Distress Index[a,f]	**[McCubbin et.al., 1996]**	**1**	**8**	**Severity of family distress**
Family Index of Regenerativity General[a,e]	**[McCubbin et.al., 1996]**	**1**	**74**	**Blends items from several scales and Adaptation - (FILE, FCOPES, SSI, FHI) to test major dimensions of resiliency model: family stressors, family strains, relative and friend support, social support, family coherence, family hardiness, family distress**
The Family Profile[a,h]	**[Sawin & Harrigan, 1995]; [Halvorsen, 1992]**	**1**	**90**	**Family concordance, family discordance, marital strength, active involvement, religiosity, parental leadership**

Table 6.1 (continued)

Family, Friends, and Self Form[a,f]	**[Simpson & McBride, 1992]**	**1**	**63**	**Family relations (warmth, control, conflict), friend relations (activity, trouble, familiar with parents, involvement), self relations (self-esteem, environment, school)**
Self Report Family Inventory[a,c]	**[Sawin & Harrigan, 1995] [Hampson et.al., 1989]**	**1**	**36**	**Health/competence, conflict, cohesion, directive leadership, expressiveness**
Family Assessment Caregiver (University of Wisconsin)[a,f]	**[Greenburg et.al, 1993]**	**1**	**21**	**Validation, family of origin, roles, problem solving, Scale boundary**
Differentiation in the Family Scale[b,g]	**[Anderson et.al., 1992]**	**1**	**11**	**Family differentiation**
Family Assessment Form[a,h]	**[McCroskey et.al., 1991]**	**1**	**102**	**Physical environment, social supports, financial environment, psychosocial history, personal characteristics, child-rearing, caregiver-child interaction**

1=English, 2=French, 3=Hungarian, 4=Dutch, 5=Portuguese, 6=Spanish, 7=Afrikaans, 8=Hebrew, 9=German,10=Puerto Rican, 11=Vietnamese, 12=Japanese, 13=Korean,14=American Sign Language, 15=Iceland, 16=Danish, 17=Swedish, 18=Finland, 19=Estonia, 20= Norway

a= reliability coefficient >.50 but <.90, b= reliability coefficient >.90, c= reliability coefficient <.50, d= validity coefficient >.60 but < .70, e= validity coefficient > .80, f= validity coefficient < .60, g= validity coefficients not reported though known groups validity did discriminate according to model's assumptions, h= no validity confirmation reported thinking, playing and working, communicating, sex, finding meaning, and transcending. The intent of the model is to "stimulate new ways of approaching personal issues or problems" (Palombi, 1992, p. 221).

The psychological well-being model has six dimensions: autonomy, environmental mastery, personal growth, positive relations with others, purpose in life, and self-acceptance. Using a telephone interview survey approach, Carol D. Ryff and Corey L. Keyes (1995) empirically confirmed the model's dimensions.

It is hoped the reader can see from the above description that the concept of wellness (and empirical measurement of the construct) can be quite diverse, depending on the model chosen. Personal growth is emphasized in one model, clinical relief in another. Table 6.2 further elaborates on the choices we have when trying to capture the concept of health or wellness.

Table 6.2 further illustrates that the range of what can be considered health, wellness, or hardiness challenges the clinician to conceptualize what she or he is trying to accomplish with families. Concepts such as health responsibility, personal growth, commitment, and spirituality are advocated as part of wellness. Few of the wellness projects have sought to expand the wellness issue to focus on family-level assessment. Few of the wellness projects explain how their model works with clients in the midst of severe disease or illness. Prevention, exercise and nutritional activity levels, and motivation to stay healthy take on a whole new meaning with a patient with advanced AIDS. Can that person (or his/her family) have a high level of wellness in spite of severe disease?

BLENDING OF FAMILY FUNCTIONING AND HEALTH/ WELLNESS MEASURES

The above list of family measures and wellness measures demonstrates that a wide range of assessment choices is available for the clinician. But how should they be blended? The family functioning measures identify dimensions that can be easily defended as measures of family health themselves. Family cohesion, problem-solving skill, affective involvement, and financial well-being are constructs that have a lot to do with family health. But wellness factors such as health responsibility, activity level, and spirituality are useful as well.

This author suggests that the best approach is to develop a combination of measures (with clear theoretical framework) that provide a more com-

Table 6.2
Measures of Well-Being, Wellness, or Health

MEASURE	SOURCE	SIZE	CONSTRUCTS
Laffrey Health Conception Scale	(Laffrey, 1986; Lusk et al, 1995)	28 or 16	Clinical health, role performance health,adaptive health, eudaimonistic (self-actualizing) health
Health-Promoting Lifestyle Profile	(Walker et al, 1987; Oleckno & Blacconiere, 1990)	48	Self-actualization, health responsibility, exercise, nutrition, interpersonal support, stress management
Lifestyle Assessment Questionnaire	(Palombi, 1992) DeStefano et al, 1992)	100	Physical fitness, nutrition, self-care, drugs and driving, environment, emotional awareness, emotional control, intellectual, occupational, spiritual
Wellness Inventory	(Travis, 1981; Palombi, 1992)	120	Self-responsibility and love, breathing, sensing, eating, moving,feeling, thinking, playing and working, communicating, sex, finding meaning, transcending
Lifestyle Coping Inventory	(Hinds, 1983; (Palombi, 1992)	142	Coping style actions, nutritional actions, physical care actions, cognitive and emotional actions, low risk actions, environmental actions, social support actions
Family Member Well-being Index	(McCubbin et al, 1996)	8	Emotional, social, interactional and physical well-being

Theoretically Grounded Scales of Psychological Well-being	**(Ryff & Keyes, 1995)**	**18**	**Self-acceptance, personal growth, purpose in life, positive relations with others, environmental mastery, autonomy**
Wellness Index	**(Slivinske & Fitch, 1992)**	**69**	**Physical health, morale, daily living activity ability, spirituality, social resources**
Hardiness Scale	**(Kobasa et al, 1982; Tartasky, 1993)**	**20**	**Commitment, control, challenge**
Health Related Hardiness Scale	**(Pollard & Duffy, 1990; Tartasky, 1993)**	**36**	**Commitment, control**
Family Hardiness Index	**(McCubbin et al; 1996)**	**20**	**Co-oriented commitment, confidence, challenges, control**

prehensive picture. Some examples might be (a) Generic Assessment Protocol and (b) Family Wellness Checkups.

Generic Assessment Protocol

INTAKE: Family Assessment Device or Family Attachment and Changeability Index to assess family functioning, Lifestyle Assessment Questionnaire for adults in family to gauge activity level and high-risk behavior.

FOLLOWUP: Family Member Well-Being Index as a quick check of family health status and FAD or FACI at periodic intervals.

Family Wellness Checkups

The clinician could designate a session as a family wellness checkup. Use Family Inventory of Life and Changes (FILC) to gauge pileup potential, Feetham Family Functioning Scale to gauge linkage between family and other systems, Family Assessment Device to assess family structure, and the Lifestyle Coping Inventory to gauge the degree of wellness activity in members. The checkup can lead to outcomes which are incorporated into a family wellness plan. In a managed care framework, the plan gives excellent parameters: outcome focus, clear direction for intervention, and a wellness emphasis.

FUTURE DIRECTIONS IN FAMILY HEALTH SOCIAL WORK PRACTICE

There are numerous ways to capitalize on the growing interest in wellness. Certainly several professions are asserting expertise (Cowen, 1991; Myers, 1991; Pardeck, Yuen, Daley, & Hawkins, 1998), and wellness approaches are being implemented in battered women's shelters (Donaghy, 1995), on college campuses (DeStefano & Harger, 1990), in elementary schools (Omizo, Omiza, & D'Andrea, 1992), and prisons (Peterson & Johnstone, 1995). Concurrently, efforts to enhance family health are increasing. Whether called family resilience (Hawley & deHaan, 1996), family preservation (Blythe, Salley, & Jayaratne, 1994), or family competence (Lewis, Beavers, Gossett, & Phillips, 1976), researchers and clinicians are increasingly advocating for a shift from pathology to wellness in intervention and assessment. In short, family health is an area with rich potential for collaboration and research.

There are many directions in which the collaboration or research could go. First, research should occur to blend the family functioning measures shown in table 6.1 and the wellness questions in table 6.2 in order to create a brief assessment scale that covers both constructs (family and health). The examples of mixing scales given in the above section are useful but impractical because of the size of the measures. The challenge would be to blend the constructs into a scale of fewer than 30 items that can be practically used as a quick gauge in session.

Second, the wellness constructs need to be clarified to allow use of measures with patients (and families) with severe physical diseases. Some of the measures are scored according to absence of disease. Wellness can occur or deteriorate in an intensive care patient. Wellness needs to capture constructs concurrent to presence or absence of physical capability.

Third, combinations of family measures and wellness measures should be tried out in wellness checkups to determine if they help the clinician assist the family better. Outcome research on utility of measures in defining family wellness status and improvement would be invaluable. Such data can help reinforce the molasses movement of the managed health care industry toward higher reimbursement of preventive activity. Specifically, reimbursement for family wellness-enhancing activity would be invaluable in institutionalizing a family focus in health care delivery.

Finally, research needs to clarify the links or conflicts between individual and family wellness. Do they rise or deteriorate concurrently? Is individual wellness an autonomous factor to family wellness? Is there a critical mass of individual wellness or health in order to achieve adequate family health, or does any member's poor health (e.g., alcoholic father) damage the family's health?

SUMMARY

It is hoped this chapter has provided more insight into some of the current models of family functioning and wellness, measures that are available for clinician use today, and future directions to consider. We have a long way to go before user-friendly family-level measurements are incorporated into every clinician's office. But beginning with what is available and demanding better clinical instruments spotlights the need.

REFERENCES

Anderson, S. A., & Sabatelli, R. M. (1992). The differentiation in the family system scale (DIFS). *American Journal of Family Therapy, 20*(1), 77–89.

Bennett, M. J. (1993). View from the bridge: Reflections of a recovering staff model HMO psychiatrist. *Psychiatric Quarterly, 64*(1), 45–75.

Bloom, M., Fischer, J., & Orme, J. G. (1995). *Evaluating practice: Guidelines for the accountable professional* (2nd ed.). Boston: Allyn and Bacon.

Blythe, B. J., Salley, M. P., & Jayaratne, S. (1994). A review of intensive family preservation services research. *Social Work Research, 18*(4), 213–224.

Brown, F. (1994). Resisting the pull of the health insurance tarbaby: An organizational model for surviving managed care. *Clinical Social Work Journal, 22*, 59–71.

Cowen, E. L. (1991). In pursuit of wellness. *American Psychologist, 46*(4), 404–408.

Cowen, E. L. (1994). The enhancement of psychological wellness: Challenges and opportunities. *American Journal of Community Psychology, 22*(2), 149–179.

Daley, J. G., & Bostock, D. J. (1998). A world view model of health care utilization: The impact of social and provider context on health care decision making. *Journal of Health and Social Policy, 9*(4), 67–82.

Daley, J. G., Sowers-Hoag, K. M., & Thyer, B. A. (1990). Are FACES-II ''family satisfaction'' scores valid? *Journal of Family Therapy, 12*, 77–81.

Daley, J. G., Sowers-Hoag, K. M., & Thyer, B. A. (1991). Construct validity of the circumplex model of family functioning. *Journal of Social Service Research, 15*(1–2), 131–147.

DeStefano, T. J., & Harger, B. (1990). Promoting the wellness life-style on a college campus. *Journal of College Student Development, 31*(5), 461–462.

DeStefano, T. J., & Richardson, P. (1992). The relationship of paper-and-pencil wellness measures to objective physiological indexes. *Journal of Counseling and Development, 71*, 226–230.

Donaghy, K. B. (1995). Beyond survival: Applying wellness interventions in battered women's shelters. *Journal of Mental Health Counseling, 17*(1), 3–17.

Dorwart, R. A. (1990). Managed mental health care: Myths and realities in the 1990s. *Hospital and Community Psychiatry, 41*(10), 1087–1091.

Eckblad, G. F. (1991). The ''circumplex'' and curvilinear functions. *Family Process, 32*(4), 473–476.

Feetham, S. L. (1991). *Feetham family functioning survey manual.* Washington, DC: Children's National Medical Center.

Fischer, J., & Corcoran, K. (1994). *Measures for clinical practice: A sourcebook.* New York: Free Press.

Frankel, P. W. (1992, November/December). Profiling ambulatory care physicians. *Journal of Health Care Benefits*, 21–24.

Green, R. G., Harris, R. N., Forte, J. A., & Robinson, M. (1991). Evaluating FACES III and the circumplex model: 2,440 families. *Family Process, 30*(1), 55–73.

Greenburg, J. R., Monson, T., & Gesino, J. (1993). Development of University of Wisconsin family assessment caregiver scale (UW-FACS): A new measure to assess families caring for a frail elderly member. *Journal of Gerontological Social Work, 19*(3/4), 49–68.

Halvorsen, J. G. (1992). The family profile: A new self-report instrument for family assessment. *Family Practice Research Journal, 12*(4), 343–367.

Hampson, R. B., Beavers, W. R., & Hulgus, Y. F. (1989). Insiders' and outsiders' views of family: The assessment of family competence and style. *Journal of Family Psychology, 3*, 118–136.

Hawley, D. R., & deHaan, L. (1996). Toward a definition of family resilience: Integrating life-span and family perspectives. *Family Process, 35*, 283–298.

Hettler, W. (1980). Wellness promotion on a university campus. *Journal of Health Promotion and Maintenance, 3*(1), 77–95.

Hinds, W. C. (1983). *Personal paradigm shift: A lifestyle intervention approach to health care management.* East Lansing: Michigan State University.

Hudson, W. W. (1982). *The clinical measurement package: A field manual.* Homewood, IL: Dorsey Press.

Hudson, W. W. (1992). *WALMYR assessment scales scoring manual.* Tempe, AZ: WALMYR.

Jensen, L. A., & Allen, M. N. (1994). A synthesis of qualitative research on wellness-illness. *Qualitative Health Research, 4*(4), 349–369.

Kobasa, S. C., Maddi, S. R., & Kahn, S. (1982). Hardiness and health: A prospective study. *Journal of Personality and Social Psychology, 42*, 168–177.

Kunnes, R. (1992). Managed mental health: The insurer's perspective. In S. Feldman (Ed.), *Managed mental health services* (pp. 101–125). Springfield, IL: Charles C. Thomas.

Laffrey, S. (1986). Development of a health conception scale. *Research in Nursing Health, 9*, 107–113.

Lasky, P., Buckwalter, K. C., Whall, W., Lederman, R., Speer, J., McClane, A., King, J. M., & White, M. A. (1985). Developing an instrument for the assessment of family dynamics. *Western Journal of Nursing Research, 7*, 40–57.

Lewis, J. M., Beavers, W. R., Gossett, J. T., & Phillips, V. A. (1976). *No single thread: Psychological health in family systems*. New York: Brunner/Mazel.

Lusk, S. L., Kerr, M. J., & Baer, L. M. (1995). Psychometric testing of the reduced Laffrey health conception scale. *American Journal of Health Promotion, 9*(3), 220–224.

McCroskey, J., Nishimoto, R., & Subramanian, K. (1991). Assessment in family support programs: Initial reliability and validity testing of the family assessment form. *Child Welfare, 70*(1), 19–33.

McCubbin, H. I., Thompson, A. I., & McCubbin, M. A. (1996). *Family assessment: Resiliency, coping and adaptation: Inventories for research and practice*. Madison: University of Wisconsin.

Miller, I. W., Bishop, D. S., Keitner, G. I., & Epstein, N. B. (in press). *The McMaster approach to families: Theory, treatment and research*. New York: Pergamon Press.

Miller, I. W., Epstein, N. B., Bishop, D. S., & Keitner, G. I. (1985). The McMaster family assessment device: Reliability and validity. *Journal of Marital and Family Therapy, 11*(4), 345–356.

Mizrahi, T. (1993). Managed care and managed competition: A primer for social work. *Health and Social Work, 18*(2), 86–91.

Moos, R. H. (1990). Conceptual and empirical approaches to developing family-based assessment procedures: Resolving the case of the Family Environmental Scale. *Family Process, 29*, 199–208.

Myers, J. E. (1991). Wellness as the paradigm for counseling and development: The possible future. *Counselor Education and Supervision, 30*(3), 183–193.

Nurius, P. S., & Hudson, W. W. (1993). *Human services practice, evaluation, and computers: A practical guide for today and beyond*. Pacific Grove, CA: Brooks/Cole.

Oleckno, W. A., & Blacconiere, M. J. (1990). Wellness of college students and differences by gender, race, and class standing. *College Student Journal, 24*(4), 421–429.

Olson, D. H. (1991). Commentary: Three dimensional (3-D) circumplex model and revised scoring of FACES III. *Family Process, 30*, 74–79.

Olson, D. H., McCubbin, H. I., Barnes, H., Larsen, A., Muxen, M., & Wilson, M. (1985). *Family inventories*. St. Paul, MN: University of Minnesota, Family Social Science.

Omizo, M. M., Omiza, S. A., & D'Andrea, M. J. (1992). Promoting wellness among elementary school children. *Journal of Counseling and Development, 71*(2), 194–198.

Palombi, B. J. (1992). Psychometric properties of wellness instruments. *Journal of Counseling and Development, 71*, 221–225.

Pardeck, J. T., Yuen, F. K. O., Daley, B., & Hawkins, K. (1998). Social work assessment and intervention through family health practice. *Family Therapy, 25*(1), 25–39.

Pender, N. (1984). Health promotion and illness prevention. *Annual Review of Nursing Research, 2*, 83–105.

Peterson, M., & Johnstone, B. M. (1995). The Atwood Hall Health Promotion Program, Federal Medical Center, Lexington, KY: Effects on drug-involved federal offenders. *Journal of Substance Abuse Treatment, 12*(1), 43–48.

Pollard, S. E., & Duffy, M. E. (1990). The health-related hardiness scale: Development and psychometric analysis. *Nursing Research, 39*, 218–222.

Ryff, C. D., & Keyes, C. L. (1995). The structure of psychological well-being revisited. *Journal of Personality and Social Psychology, 69*(4), 719–727.

Sawin, K. J., & Harrigan, M. P. (1995). *Measures of family functioning for research and practice*. New York: Springer.

Simpson, D. D., & McBride, A. A. (1992). Family, friends, and self (FFS) assessment for Mexican American youth. *Hispanic Journal of Behavioral Sciences, 14*(3), 327–340.

Skinner, H. A. (1987). Self-report instruments for family assessment. In T. Jacob (Ed.), *Family interaction and psychopathology* (pp. 172–185). New York: Plenum.

Slivinske, L. R., & Fitch, V. L. (1992). The effect of health care coverage on medical cost, utilization and well-being of the aged. *Journal of Health and Social Policy, 4*(1), 1–11.

Smith, J. (1981). The idea of health: A philosophical inquiry. *Advances in Nursing Sciences, 3*, 43–51.

Tartasky, D. S. (1993). Hardiness: Conceptual and methodological issues. *IMAGE: Journal of Nursing Scholarship, 25*(3), 225–229.

Travis, J. W. (1981). *The wellness inventory*. Mill Valley, CA: Wellness Associates.

Walker, S. N., Sechrist, K. R., & Pender, N. J. (1987). The health-promoting lifestyle profile: Development and psychometric characteristics. *Nursing Research, 36*(2), 76–81.

Zimpfer, D. G. (1992). Psychosocial treatment of life-threatening disease: A wellness model. *Journal of Counseling and Development, 71*, 203–209.

7

Family Health and Cultural Diversity

Francis K. O. Yuen

The family health social work approach considers culture and cultural diversity as integral parts of its theoretical and practice frameworks. Although different cultures have specific meanings and practice for the notion of health and family, the attainment of the well-being of the family and its members appears to be a common goal across cultures.

Cultural diversity in social work is based on the idea that the United States is a multicultural society and that different cultural beliefs and practices should be taken into consideration in social work interventions. This orientation of cultural relativity supports the notion that there is no "one size fits all" social work assessment and intervention approach. Instead, interventions have to be tailored to fit the clients' cultural context; clients' perceptions and meanings of events and issues, along with other personal, social, economic, and environmental factors, play important roles in the formation and implementation of social work interventions. Human diversity or cultural diversity calls for social workers to formulate differential and culturally appropriate interventions in working with clients of diverse backgrounds.

In general usage, cultural diversity, cultural pluralism, and multiculturalism are terms that are used almost interchangeably. Practically and academically, each has specific connotations. Cultural diversity, also referred to as human diversity, suggests the acknowledgment of the existence of people of different cultures. People who accept cultural diversity do not remain culturally apathetic and become aware of different cultures. Cultural pluralism implies the recognition, intention, and practice of working with people with different backgrounds. It involves the growth from cultural awareness to cultural sensitivity and the ability to effectively communicate cross-culturally. Multiculturalism not only recognizes differences and similarities among diverse cultures but also requires a framework of thinking that is inclusive and transcultural. This framework requires the ability to develop beyond cultural sensitivity to the level of cultural competency in interacting with people of various backgrounds. It requires one to think and act not only from the ethnic specific perspective but also from a multiple and collective perspective that allows one to conceive common good and understanding.

The idea of cultural diversity and the development of multiculturalism have generated many academic, social, and political discussions in the past decades. While most have embraced the values of diversity and strive to become more competent in working with clients of different backgrounds, some have questioned it as merely a movement of political correctness that overrepresents the minority perspective.

SOCIAL WORK EDUCATION AND HUMAN DIVERSITY

Social work has a long history of working with people whose backgrounds differ from that of the majority population. The inclusion of diversity in social work education, however, is relatively recent (Gould, 1995; Johnson, 1995). The Council on Social Work Education (CSWE) 1994 Curriculum Policy Standards require all accredited social work programs to have content on human diversity as one of nine required curriculum content areas (Council on Social Work Education [CSWE], 1994). The goal of this content is to help students understand and appreciate human diversity. Social work programs must provide content about differences and similarities in the experiences, needs, and beliefs of diverse people. Under these 1994 Curriculum Policy Standards, human diversity is defined in a broad fashion. Diversity includes groups distinguished by race, ethnicity, culture, class, gender, sexual orientation, religion, physical or mental ability, age, and national origin. In essence, human diversity is an all-inclusive concept that includes many different categories of people.

In 1984, the CSWE Curriculum Policy Standards had a much narrower view, where human diversity was included under the Special Populations curriculum content area (CSWE, 1984). Social work programs were to include course content on people of color and women. Programs could also focus on other oppressed groups if they so desired; however, there was not a specific standard that dealt solely with human diversity. The result of these earlier standards was that most programs simply focused on people of color in human diversity courses (Gould, 1995). The content of such courses on the topic of diversity was primarily tailored to fit the needs of the dominant group of white social work students. The belief was that this approach would help enable those white students to better engage in ethnic-sensitive practice. In reality, a one-directional model of teaching about pluralism was created which at best taught students to look at, rather than into, the lives of people of color (Gould, 1995). Jim Lantz and Karen V. Harper (1989) and Harper and Lantz (1996) even suggested that this model did not work, was not useful, and may have, in fact, done damage to minority clients.

Karen V. Harper and Jim Lantz (1996) conclude that a more enlightened view of human diversity should be grounded in cross-cultural social work practice. This approach to curriculum content on human diversity is designed to help students accept and respect human differences and respect human similarities. Even though the new CSWE 1994 Curriculum Policy standards stress this approach to human diversity, few social work programs have incorporated this important material into their current curriculum on diversity (Sowers-Hoag & Sander-Bechler, 1996).

ECOSYSTEMS PERSPECTIVE AND DIVERSITY

The family health social work approach, which emphasizes ecological and systems (ecosystems) orientations, views diversity as the inherent part of every ecosystem, including the family and its members. Diversity is part of the source, process, and outcome of any live ecosystem. From an ecosystems perspective, individual and family as "habitats" occupy particular "niches" in the environment; their existence and "reciprocal exchanges" with others form the "relatedness" as well as the life experience of rewards and difficulties. Individuals and families develop particular "coping" strategies, meaningful to their culture and reality, to deal with various life "stresses" throughout the individual and family life cycles. The environments in which they reside behave either as closed systems that will eventually become extinct or as open systems that require continuous input, output, and feedback to thrive. These environments also interact and network constantly with other ecosystems. Family health–centered social work practitioners should understand the dynamics of these networks in order to provide proper interventions.

Louise C. Johnson (1995, p. 138) outlines factors that social workers may use to understand clients from a particular culture. These factors are grouped into (a) cultural factors, (b) dominant societal attitudes and behaviors, and (c) individual differences. Cultural factors include values, relationship, family structure, history, communication pattern, community structure, and coping mechanism.

Factors related to dominant societal attitudes and behaviors include discrimination and stratification, ethnic consciousness, relationship to majority culture, quality of life issues, group identity and expectations of a group relative to the majority group, the ways in which difference is valued, and opportunity provision or restriction.

Individual differences include orientation to tradition and assimilation, attitude toward self and others, self-concept, coping and adaptation mechanisms, relationship with family and/or cultural groups as well as responsibility or resources in the relationship, significant life experiences as a member of the cultural group, and dynamics of self affected by diverse status. This framework provides a useful tool for social workers to understand the interactions and dynamics between individuals and their social and cultural environments.

As previously discussed, from an ecosystems perspective, family and individual reality makes up the niche for the family and individuals. This niche may be a positive one that promotes self-image or a negative one that reinforces prejudice and devaluation. Oppressed groups and minorities have long experienced discrimination and devaluation. They have used various means to cope with these stresses and to make sense of or give meaning to their often-adverse realities. Unfortunately, some of these devaluations are internalized, negatively affecting the development of the definition of self. The effects that oppression and discrimination have on the perception of reality by minority clients should be an essential part of all assessments and interventions. Similarly, the effective use of empowerment and advocacy should therefore be the integral part of any intervention.

Additional intervention concerns should include the identification of stresses and the development of culturally and developmentally appropriate coping strategies and skills. The goals of family health social work interventions are to restore, maintain, or achieve the holistic wellness of the individual and the family.

SOCIAL CONSTRUCTIVIST AND CROSS-CULTURAL PRACTICE

The social constructivist perspective is also a part of the theoretical orientations of the family health approach. This approach values the client's search for meaning and assumes that reality is socially constructed. Reality is not discovered; instead it is constructed through social interactions. Part of the role of a social worker or therapist is to honor the clients' perspectives, introduce "novelty" or new alternative views to the client systems, and coconstruct a new and meaningful reality. Cynthia Franklin and Paula S. Nurius (1996) summarize the general assumptions among social constructivists: "(1) humans actively participate in the construction of the reality to which they respond; (2) cognition, affect, and behavior exist in an interactive system; (3) life-span development is important; and (4) internal cognitive (including affective) structures such as core ordering process, deep structure, meaning systems, and narrative (life stories) are important in maintaining and changing behavior" (pp. 323–324).

Gilbert J. Greene, Carla Jensen, and Dorothy H. Jones (1996) emphasize the important use of self and the understanding of different worldviews in cross-cultural practice from a social constructivist perspective. They further assert that social workers who work with diverse clients should first develop a sense of comfort in their own ethnic and cultural self or identity. The development of self, according to Salvator Minuchin (1979), is closely affected by the family of origin which provides the context for development. Similarly, the development of the reality for the family is affected by the family's cultural heritage and its social context. It is necessary for social workers to become cognizant of the influence of family and culture for their clients and for themselves.

Hilary N. Weaver (1998) identifies human service providers' knowledge of the culture group, their ability to be self-reflective and recognize bias, and their ability to integrate knowledge and reflection with practice skills as the three main principles for service providers to become culturally competent. Adopting from T. Real's (1990) framework, Greene, Jensen, and Jones (1996) further promote the use of different stances that include eliciting, reframing, contextualizing, matching, and amplifying in facilitating diverse clients to construct and repair their realities.

The family health social work approach recognizes that the way in which one perceives reality will affect the definition of problems and the identification of alternatives and interventions. A problem situation for one person in one culture or in one particular environment may not be a problem for another person in another culture or environment. An individual's worldview dictates how one defines and approaches different situations. Worldview is, essentially, how one believes that the world works, a personal epistemology. It provides the framework for individuals to perceive and construct their personal daily reality.

Allie C. Kilpatrick and Thomas P. Holland (1995) conclude that the social constructivist approach to family practice emphasizes the strength, rather than the pathology, of the individual and the family. The focus is on the discovery of the commonalties and capacity of individuals and their families. "Family functioning is dependent upon coherent and integrated patterns of meaning, shared by all the members" (p. 28). Similarly, "diversity issues must be recognized with the goal of developing mutual respect and appreciation for differences" (p. 49). Social constructivists focus on the commonalties that unite people, not the differences that divide them. The basic expectation of a family health social worker, who integrates the social constructivist orientation, is to listen and learn professionally and form a "therapeutic alliance" with the clients. The worker then facilitates a client to become an active author of the culturally appropriate new reality that addresses the situation in question.

ACCULTURATION AND SOURCE OF KNOWLEDGE

Charles R. Atherton and David L. Klemmack (1982) list four sources of knowledge: tradition, experience, common sense, and scientific knowledge. Tradition is customs and beliefs that have been handed down from generation to generation. It is not necessarily logical or rational, but it makes sense to the people who practice it. Experience is the person's firsthand observation. Siblings of the same family may share the same family or cultural tradition, but their different personal observations of events in the family and in their lives make them distinctly different individuals. Experience is unique and sometimes can only be understood by the individuals involved.

Common sense is a difficult concept to define because everyone assumes it is so common that everyone knows what it is. Technically, common sense is the combination of tradition and experience. Obviously, what is common sense for one person may not be for another person, particularly if the two people have different traditions and experiences. Scientific knowledge is developed mainly through logical and rational validations. It is not the source of absolute knowledge, but it provides the objective means of knowing in addition to the other more subjective ways of knowing.

For example, an elderly woman in the neighborhood is a well-known do-gooder. She knows the tradition well and has seen many events in her life. She has a great common sense of how things are coming about and how they will go. She is therefore well respected by the people in the community; they view her as a source of wisdom. However, she may not know how to go about providing help in a professional manner that is often grounded in scientific knowledge. Conversely, a well-educated social worker who has a doctoral degree in social work may possess the scientific and professional knowledge, but his or her lack of common sense, particularly in relation to that community, makes professional training and helping skills seem out of touch with the community. A culturally competent social worker, therefore, is one who can apply his/her professional knowledge and skills in a manner that makes sense within the client system. This results in a professional practice that can be understood by clients based on their tradition, experience, common sense, and education.

People of different backgrounds come to America via different routes and have different experiences of their receptions in America. Service providers should be aware of the several types of cultures that may affect their practice, particularly with new immigrants: native/ethnic culture, clients' migration and minority status experience, new cultures that are formed by the immigrants and their children, the local/American culture and view of diversity, and the service providers' personal cultural background.

By tabulating the type of knowledge versus the type of culture, one can easily see the web of possible realities involved in any cross-cultural intervention (see table 7.1). A traditional (native and ethnic) Vietnamese refugee father who risked his life and suffered many hardships to bring his family to the United States (migration and minority experience) and lives in a rather homogeneous and conservative mid-American town (local majority American) will have a difficult time working with a young black social worker who has very limited exposure to anything other than black and white cultures (service provider's culture) about the father's American-born daughter's desire to move out of the home, supporting herself through part-time work while completing her fine arts degree and raising her out-of-wedlock baby (new culture). The interactions among these possible realities also creates another dynamic, while sometime chaotic, environment in which a social worker must navigate

Table 7.1
Types of Knowledge and Cultural Differences

	Immigrants' or Minorities'			Local's or Majority's	
	Native or Ethnic Culture	Migration or Minority Status Experience	New Cultures	Local or Majority Americans' Culture	Service Providers' Culture
Traditions	Native traditions	Migration or minority traditions	New traditions	Local or majority traditions	Service providers' traditions
Experiences	Native experiences	Migration or minority experiences	New experiences	Local or majority experiences	Service providers' experiences
Common Senses	Native common sense	Migration or minority common senses	New common senses	Local or majority common senses	Service providers' common senses
Scientific Knowledge	Native knowledge	Migration or minority knowledge	New knowledge	Local or majority knowledge	Service providers' knowledge

and purposefully move the family and its members toward a desirable state of well-being.

While it is impossible for service providers to become familiar with all types of culture and know the exact level of acculturation of their clients, it is possible for workers to acknowledge the clients' different viewpoints and facilitate changes within the clients, their families, and their social environments. Workers who have a static ''cultural boundary'' will be ineffective in providing service cross-culturally. Equally important is the worker's well-grounded and anchored self-awareness and acceptance of his/her own cultural identity.

CULTURALLY COMPETENT FAMILY HEALTH PRACTICE

A culturally competent family health–centered social work practice operating within the theoretical framework of family health should also consider the following factors:

1. Accessibility, availability, and acculturation.
2. Utilization and identification of effective point of entry.
3. Extensive contacts in a client's environment to allow the building of a productive working relationship.

4. Family as well as the individual as the units of intervention.
5. Culturally appropriate assessment and intervention procedures.

Accessibility refers to both geographical and cultural relevance as well as difficulties in service delivery. Ideally, the service delivery location is within reach of the target population. Transportation is a common barrier that keeps clients, particularly new immigrants and minorities, from getting services. Furthermore, whether clients can culturally and linguistically access or communicate with the service provider often determines their desire to use the service. Local or bicultural and bilingual workers who are respected by their ethnic or minority community are vital to bridge this gap.

Availability refers to the existence, recruitment, and retention of service, clients, and qualified service providers. It is a factor that is closely related to accessibility. Family health social workers not only should be resourceful in linking clients to existing services; they should also advocate for needed services, empower clients to fully utilize appropriate services, and prepare for qualified and culturally competent service providers. In some minority communities, the proper use of paraprofessionals and local formal and informal support networks are effective means to make services available to the communities.

For example, a relatively large number of Cambodian refugees arrived in the United States and particularly in California in the late 1970s. Many of them were women and children who were separated from their families. Many were traumatized by the wars and genocide from which they just escaped. Because educated and professional Cambodian refugees destroyed any traces of their education and training during the wars in order to save their lives, there were no "qualified" Cambodian health and human service professionals who could serve that community.

Concerned service providers and Cambodian social activists advocated fiercely to gain funding support to develop Southeast Asian–specific services. They hired leaders from the various Cambodian neighborhoods to provide an array of needed services from resettlement to health and mental health interventions. These community leaders were provided with intensive training on health and mental health interventions and were closely supervised by or paired with another Asian-American human service professional. Without these paraprofessionals, the health and mental health needs of the Cambodian communities would have gone unnoticed and unserved by the existing service systems.

Acculturation refers to the quality and extent of exposure to the dominant American culture and the degree of social functioning within the dominant culture. Differential assessments of clients' extent of acculturation help locate the locus of concerns and the most appropriate interventions for the client. E. R. Oetting and Fred Beauvais (1990–91) and Oetting (1993) suggest that individuals who have low cultural identification will have more difficulty in performing behaviors that are culturally congruent. They are likely to be forced to turn to other subcultures to meet their needs and may become involved in some high-risk behaviors such as substance abuse and criminal involvement.

Meanwhile, certain individuals may choose to identify with their traditional ethnic culture or the new host culture. These individuals may be comfortable with continuing to be traditional in their way of life or may totally immerse themselves into the host culture and adopt it as their own. Although these two groups may be at the two extremes in terms of acculturation, in reality, both groups have a firm identification with a particular culture. This firm identity has served as a resiliency factor in dealing with many life events. Bicultural individuals are those who can function effectively within both the old and new cultures and are considered culturally successful. On the opposite side, anomic people are those who cannot identify with either the old or the new host culture. The conditions of normlessness make them more likely to experience difficulties in dealing with life issues.

Different clients have different degrees of readiness in approaching and receiving service from service providers. Culturally, there are different help- or care-seeking beliefs and behaviors. James W. Green (1995) asserts that care is a cultural concept that is socially constructed and implies a worldview of preference. Care is also a system of communication and disclosure including language, procedure, and styles or mannerisms that are known and meaningful to the people within the community. Receiving or giving help or care, therefore, can be a ritualistic process that carries tremendous significance to the recipients as well as the community. In many cultures, help seeking is both a community and an individual issue.

The family health social worker should be sensitive to this subtle but significant consideration. A comprehensive service center that provides an array of related services and is located in the neighborhood is an example of such "one-stop" service locations. These agencies provide a convenient and less-stigmatized environment for clients, and often the whole family, to access and receive referral for services. The reputations of the service organization and its workers play a major role in clients' decision of whether to come for services. It implies the degree of trust, confidence, and acceptance that clients have toward the service providers and the organizations.

Once clients approach the service organizations, a family health social worker not only should address the immediate concerns or crises of the clients, he/she should also assist the client in placing the situation within the larger context, including the family environment. The assessment and intervention techniques again have to be linguistically and culturally appropriate. A reverent relationship between an Asian elderly mother and her daughter or a protective relationship between two teen Hispanic brothers may be seen as codependent relationships in the traditional clinical assessment. Culturally it may be the kind of interdependence that has sustained these minority families in times of crisis and need.

Harper and Lantz (1996) identified eight "cross-cultural curative factors" that may aid social workers in developing culturally appropriate interventions with diverse client populations:

1. Worldview Respect: Effective healing and healing methods have to be compatible with clients' worldview.
2. Hope: Greater hope that the clients have toward the intervention process and its outcome is likely to lead to clients' greater improvement.
3. Helper Attractiveness: Clients' perception of the service practitioner's ability to help and personal attributes.
4. Control: Develop the mastery of control through learning, empowerment, insight, self-management, and self-control.
5. Rites of Initiation: Use of appropriate rituals symbolizes life transitions from death (old behaviors) to rebirth (new behaviors). The Alcoholics Anonymous 12-step program is one such example.
6. Cleansing Experience: Sweating, confession, restitution, giving talks, community services, and catharsis are examples of rituals that deal with the recognition of human imperfection.
7. Existential Realization: Facilitate reflections that help clients discover, create, and expand meaning in their lives and challenge their existential vacuum.
8. Physical Intervention: Use of medical or biochemical treatments.

TOWARD A MULTICULTURAL PARADIGM

It is unrealistic to expect service providers to know all things about all cultures. However, it is reasonable to expect them to develop a multicultural perspective. This perspective is more than cultural pluralism, which accepts that many cultures coexist in our society. It requires a new paradigm shift—one that Ketayun H. Gould suggests changes from "viewing multiculturalism as merely a 'practice' extension of the minority perspective to a framework that can help all groups in society orient their thinking at a transcultural level" (1995, p. 203). Developing and applying this transcultural ability in order to achieve the well-being of the clients and their families is a challenge for family health social workers. This challenge calls for a genuine acceptance, respect, and utilization of what the clients have brought to the table. Through professionally guided interventions, the social worker assists the clients to reconstruct a more desirable story and a more functional reality. It is a cooperative relationship between the clients and the worker.

As Emma R. Gross (1995) puts it, "the client and social worker have each other's perceptions and resources to work with and nothing more" (p. 212). Starting with what the clients and the worker have and skillfully expanding resources and opportunities toward the goal of well-being for the family and its members in a culturally appropriate manner is rather a challenging journey of becoming than a state of unachievable being.

REFERENCES

Atherton, C., & Klemmack, D. (1982). *Research methods in social work.* Lexington, MA: D. C. Heath.

Council on Social Work Education. (1984). *Handbook of accreditation standards and procedures* (revised July 1984). Washington, DC: Author.

Council on Social Work Education. (1994). *Handbook of accreditation standards and procedures* (4th ed.). Washington, DC: Author.

Franklin, S., & Nurius, P. (1996). Editorial notes/Constructivist therapy: New directions in social work practice. *Families in Society, 77*(6), 323–325.

Gould, K. H. (1995). The misconstructing of multiculturalism: The Stanford debate and social work. *Social Work, 40*(2), 198–205.

Green, J. (1995). *Cultural awareness in the human services: A multi-ethnic approach.* Needham Heights, MA: Allyn and Bacon.

Greene, G., Jensen, C., & Jones D. (1996). A constructivist perspective on clinical social work practice with ethnically diverse clients. *Social Work, 41*(2), 172–180.

Gross, E. R. (1995). Deconstructing politically correct practice literature: The American Indian case. *Social Work, 40*(2), 206–213.

Harper, K. V., & Lantz, J. (1996). *Cross-cultural practice: Social work with diverse populations*. Chicago, IL: Lyceum Books.

Johnson, L. (1995). *Social work practice: A generalist approach* (5th ed.). Needham Heights, MA: Allyn and Bacon.

Kilpatrick, A. C., & Holland, T. P. (1995). *Working with families: An integrative model by level of functioning*. Needham Heights, MA: Allyn and Bacon.

Lantz, J., & Harper, K. (1989). Network intervention, existential depression and the relocated Appalachian family. *Contemporary Therapy, 11*, 213–223.

Leigh, J. (1983). The black experience with health care delivery systems: A focus on the practitioners. In A. E. Johnson (Ed.), *The black experience: Considerations for health and human services* (pp. 115–129). Davis, CA: International Dialogue Press.

Minuchin, S. (1979). Constructing a therapeutic reality. In E. Kaufman & P. Kaufman (Eds.), *Family therapy of drug and alcohol abuse* (pp. 5–18). Boston: Allyn and Bacon.

Oetting, E. (1993). Ortogonal cultural identification: Theoretical links between culture identification and substance. In M. De La Rosa & J. Adrados (Eds.), *Drug abuse among minority youth: Methodological issues and recent research advances* (National Institute on Drug Abuse Research Monograph 130; NIH Publication No. 93–3479). Washington, DC: Government Printing Office.

Oetting, E., & Beauvais, F. (1990–91). Orthogonal cultural identification theory: The cultural identification of minority adolescents. *International Journal of the Addictions, 25*(5A & 6A), 655–685.

Real, T. (1990). The therapeutic use of self in constructivist/systemic therapy. *Family Process, 29*, 255–272.

Sowers-Hoag, K. M., & Sander-Bechler, J. A. (1996). Educating for cultural competence in the generalist curriculum. *Journal of Multicultural Social Work, 4*, 37–56.

Weaver, H. N. (1998). Indigenous people in a multicultural society: Unique issues for human services. *Social Work, 43*(3), 203–211.

8

Family Health and Family Violence

Joan C. McClennen

Violence is an American tradition (Hay & Jones, 1994). ''Violence is the ultimate attempt to control'' (Kivel, 1992, p. 133). Violence is power; violence works (Hay & Jones; Walker, 1979).

The American family has been described as the most violent of institutions (McKay, 1994). Knowing that Susan Smith drowned her own two sons, ''it was too much to hope that [Michael and Alex] never felt the water, or the sinking, or the terror of dying together, alone'' (Gibbs, 1994, p. 43). Seven-week-old Devlin Binnings was hospitalized with shaken-baby syndrome. Apparently, the baby had urinated on his father (Wade, 1997). Dina Sorichetti, attacked by her estranged husband, was found slashed from head to toe, inflicted with internal injuries; he also attempted to saw off her leg (Jones, 1994). What persons, reading of ordinary people committing the unthinkable, have not ''worried about their own capacity for violence?'' (Gibbs, p. 44).

John T. Pardeck and Francis K. O. Yuen (1997) refer to a family as a system of two or more interacting persons who are committed for the common purpose of promoting the holistic well-being of each of its members. An epidemic is annihilating families, festering at each and every dimension of its well-being. The epidemic is family violence (Jones, 1994; Schornstein, 1997).

This chapter provides definitions, prevalence, historical perspectives, dynamics, theoretical underpinnings, correlates, policies, and prevention/intervention strategies related to intrafamilial child abuse and partner abuse.

CHILD ABUSE

Prevalence and Definition

Approximately six children are reported abused and neglected in America every minute. A child is murdered every three hours, totaling 1,200 children a year dying as a result of physical abuse or neglect. Annually, approximately three million children are abused in the United States (National Victim Center, 1995). "In 1990, the U.S. Advisory Board of Child Abuse and Neglect declared abuse a national emergency" (Dhooper & Schneider, 1995, p. 36).

Child abuse "is any physical injury, sexual abuse, or emotional abuse inflicted on a child other than by accidental means by those responsible for the child's care, custody, and control" (Child Abuse and Neglect Laws, 1996, p. 4). Recognition of the indicators of child abuse and neglect assists professionals and laypersons to fulfill their responsibility in protecting children suffering from abuse or neglect. Wallace (1996) and Ola W. Barnett, Cindy L. Miller-Perrin, and Robin D. Perrin (1997) provide detailed explanations, with accompanying pictorial depictions, of various types of abuse (physical, emotional, and sexual) and neglect including sibling abuse, nonorganic failure to thrive, and ritualistic abuse.

Historical Perspective

Viewing childhood as a special time in individuals' lives is a relatively recent concept. Historically, children were considered by society as chattel, at the mercy of their caregivers, and beyond the interference of outsiders. Plato (428 B.C.E.) and Aristotle (348 B.C.E.) urged killing of infants born with birth defects. In biblical times, King Herod ordered infanticide. In the Middle Ages children were mutilated to make them more effective beggars. During the Industrial Revolution children were beaten, shackled, and starved to force them to work harder (Barnett et al., 1997; Wallace, 1996).

The first case of child abuse receiving legal recognition occurred in 1874. Mary Ellen Wilson was found by Etta Wheeler tied to a bed, covered with scissors cuts and whip slashes. As no laws existed to protect children from caregivers' abuse, "the American Society for the Prevention of Cruelty to Animals argued in court that the child was covered under laws barring the barbaric treatment of animals" (Cohn, 1992, p. 89).

Almost 100 years passed after Mary Ellen was called to the public's attention before the American society would take a notable stride in recognizing and accepting the need for protection of abused children. In 1960, Dr. C. H. Kemp published his article in the American Medical Association (AMA) on the Battered Child Syndrome, a diagnosis applicable to any child suffering certain types of injuries over a period of time not caused by accidental means. In 1974, the federal government passed the Child Abuse and Neglect Act establishing Children's Protective Services (CPS), mandated reporting, and toll-free hotlines.

Legal Procedures

Although variations exist for procedures followed by CPS, federal laws and statutes provide guidelines for court procedures. Workers have 24 to 72 hours to investigate a reported case. If a child is taken into "temporary protective custody," a detention hearing is held before the court within 24 hours to determine sufficient cause for this action (Child Abuse and Neglect Laws, 1996, p. 7). Within 30 days an adjudicatory hearing is held at which time a preponderance of evidence is required to be presented for the judge to declare the child a "dependent," meaning "in need of the court's protection from the child's caregiver." The child usually is represented by a guardian ad litem who is an adult professional trained to speak on behalf of the child's best interest (Child Abuse and Neglect Laws, p. 18). If the child is adjudicated dependent, the court has another 30 days to determine the disposition of the child's custody. These proceedings are in civil court and are separate from any criminal proceedings against the perpetrator for the child's mistreatment.

All 50 states have mandated reporting laws and toll-free hotlines for individuals to anonymously report suspected abuse (Wallace, 1996). Professionals holding positions with responsibility for the care of children's welfare are both legally and morally responsible to report and discontinue child abuse and neglect. Callers making reports in good faith are protected by law from prosecution, and their names are confidential to the child protection agency personnel. Mandated reporters are health care professionals (physicians, medical examiners, coroners, dentists, chiropractors, optometrists, podiatrists, nurses, hospital clinic personnel), social workers, child care workers, criminal justice personnel (probation and parole officers, law enforcement officials, juvenile officers), therapists, and school personnel (Child Abuse and Neglect Laws, 1996).

Theories and Correlates of Abuse

The prevailing question as to the rationale for an adult caregiver to abuse or neglect a child remains unanswered. Barnett, Miller-Perrin, and Perrin (1997) and Harvey Wallace (1996) provide a variety of theories explaining this anomaly framed under three basic models:

1. Psychopathological Model, including the Psychopathology, Substance Abuse, and Attachment Theories.
2. Sociopsychological Model, including the Social Learning, Exchange, Cycle of Violence, and Frustration-Aggression Theories.
3. Sociocultural Model, including the Culture of Violence, Patriarchy, and General Systems Theories.

The family health practice perspective would attribute this psychologically and socially ill behavior "as an adaptive function for the family . . . maintained by family transactions and interactions . . . understood as a barometer of the pressure currently being felt within a family system" (Pardeck & Yuen, 1997, p. 126). Based on this perspective, "a holistic orientation to assessment and intervention" is required for successful intervention (Pardeck & Yuen, p. 127).

Several major surveys have been conducted on factors related to physical abuse of children including a description of the distribution of violence, the changing nature of the violence, prevention and treatment resources, and identification of high-risk groups. "One profile is based on official report data (American Association for Protecting Children [AAPC], 1986) and two are based on self-report survey data (National Center of Child Abuse and Neglect [NCCAN], 1988; and Gelles, 1980)" (Wolfner & Gelles, 1993, p. 198). Two other sources profiling violence toward children are the First National Family Violence Survey conducted in 1975 and the Second National Family Violence Survey conducted in 1985 (Wolfner & Gelles).

The data from these surveys, in addition to other empirical findings, report correlates of abusive parents: (a) insecure childhoods; (b) histories of psychological problems; (c) histories of criminal or suicidal behaviors; (d) addiction to drugs or alcohol; (e) isolation from friends and relatives; (f) emotional or financial stresses; (g) consistent illness including the Munchausen syndrome, characterized by repeated presentations for medical treatment for no apparent reason; (h) unrealistic expectations of children's developmental capacity; (i) emotional immaturity; (j) illegitimate or unwanted pregnancies; (k) presence of stepparent in home; (l) single-parent households; and (m) child's sleeping in parents' bedroom (Barnett et al., 1997; Dhooper & Schneider, 1995; Hay & Jones, 1994; Jasinski, Williams, & Brewster, 1997; Shorkey, 1979; Wallace, 1996).

Costs of Abuse

"Billions of dollars are spent each year to deal with the consequences of [child] abuse and neglect" (Sanders & Becker-Lausen, 1995, p. 272). Costs are for law enforcement, the courts, and out-of-home care as well as the medical and emotional treatment of all members of the family. Societal costs for child maltreatment also include substance abuse, adolescent pregnancy, juvenile delinquency, depression, suicide, prostitution, and violent crimes committed by victims as a result of their mistreatment as children (Miller, Veltkamp, & Janson, 1987; Orten & Rich, 1988). "It is argued that these personal and social costs far exceed the projected costs of a coordinated system of child abuse and prevention and early intervention services" (Ashford, 1994, p. 272).

Prevention and Intervention Programs

If they are to be effective, prevention and intervention programs need to assume a "family health practice approach to assessment and intervention . . . attend[ing] to not only biological factors, but also the person, the family, the community, and the social context of the person-in-the environment" (Pardeck & Yuen, 1997, pp. 125–126). "Perhaps, the most frequent and persistently noted structural factor contributing to elevated risk of maltreatment is poverty, with emphasis on certain groups among the poor—single parents, young caregivers, and those with young children" (Hay & Jones, 1994, p. 382). "Aggregate data across the 18 countries indicate that homicide of children under 14 is most closely related to a country's low level of welfare spending and a high rate of female participation in the workforce. Divorce rate is the greatest risk factor for victims over 14'' (Hay & Jones, p. 392). To be effective, prevention and intervention programs must address increased parental stress, social isolation, and residence in communities with limited resources; programs must provide job guarantees, child care, and affordable health care (Hay & Jones; Wallace, 1996).

''In the 1980s there was a virtual explosion of publications on treating the consequences of various abusive situations'' (Ashford, 1994, p. 281). Programs focusing on children find the school setting to be effective in educating children on protective measures (Dhooper & Schneider, 1995). Based on the different cognitive developmental stages throughout children's educational experience, the California Prevention and Treatment Act proposed to give all children ages 2½ to 18 an opportunity to participate in prevention training five times throughout their school careers—preschool, kindergarten, early elementary grades, junior high, and high school (Ashford, 1994). Intervention focusing on children consists of a wide range of strategies including therapeutic day treatment, play sessions, relaxation skills, problem-solving strategies, anger management, self-esteem improvement, cognitive restructuring, assertiveness training, values clarification, fair fighting, and crisis intervention techniques (Barnett et al., 1997; Blythe, 1983; Kolko, 1996; Shorkey, 1979).

A preponderance of literature regarding intervention strategies focuses on the sexually abused child. As denial and repression are primary defenses of young children, assessment and intervention is difficult (Damon, Todd, & MacFarlane, 1987). Most programs treating sexually abused children use a multimodal approach that may use a combination of any of the following: role play, sand tray, pictures or drawing of children, puppets and dolls, cognitive restructuring, guided imagery, and fantasy play. The most consistently recommended strategies provide group therapy and convince the child that the abuse was not his/her fault (Barnett et al., 1997; Cheung, Stevenson, & Leung, 1991; Grubbs, 1994; Hiebert-Murphy, De Luca, & Runtz, 1992; Himelein & McElrath, 1996; Knittle & Tuana, 1980; Lamb, 1986; Miller et al., 1987; Nelson, Miner, Marques, Russell, & Achterkirchen, 1989; Orten & Rich, 1988; Powell & Wagner, 1991; Sink, 1988; Waterman & Lusk, 1993; Winton, 1990).

Efforts to provide prevention and treatment programs have met with inconsistent findings. Ray E. Helfer (1991) proposes various impediments in prevention and intervention systems as (a) confused organizational structure, (b) movement from holistic to narrow child protection services, (c) changes from civil toward criminal handling, (d) lack of standards for state programs, (e) limited ability for professionals to problem solve together, (f) territoriality, (g) lack of national priority for children and families, (h) limited availability of treatment programs, (i) the look for the quick fix, and (j) minimal support of prevention programs.

Most importantly, effective prevention and intervention strategies "must involve entire communities and mobilize all its resources to make comprehensive changes in the support of families and the value placed on children" (Hay & Jones, 1994, p. 396). Effective preventive efforts require the commitment of every individual, family, organization, community, and governmental level (Hay & Jones).

DOMESTIC VIOLENCE: PARTNER ABUSE

Definition and Prevalence

> They are run over by cars and trucks. They have their teeth knocked out with hammers. They are raped . . . with hot curling irons. They are stabbed with knives, with ice picks, with screwdrivers. They are punched and kicked. They are burned with cigarette lighters, with cigarettes. . . . They are beaten and tortured in front of their children. . . . [Sara Buel, prosecutor] wasn't reading from an Amnesty International report. She was speaking of domestic violence. (English, 1992, p. 5)

One woman is subject to domestic violence every 13 seconds (National Clearinghouse for the Defense of Battered Women [NCHDBW], 1994, p. 98). The United States lost 39,000 soldiers in the line of duty during the Vietnam War, while during the same time period (1967–1973) 17,500 American women and children were killed by members of their families (NCHDBW, p. 96). There are more victims of domestic violence, living and dead, than there are AIDS victims, living and dead, in the United States (NCHDBW, p. 98).

Data on violence against women indicate that 20% to 25% of the adult women in the United States—between 12 and 15 million women—have been physically abused at least once by a male intimate (NCHDBW, p. 100). Each day in this country approximately four women are killed by a male intimate partner (p. 20). Domestic violence is the leading cause of injury to women, accounting for more visits to hospital emergency rooms than car crashes, muggings, and rapes combined (p. 218).

The term *domestic violence* has traditionally referred to violence between a man and woman who are involved in an intimate relationship. Pardeck and Yuen's (1997) definition provides a more inclusive basis for family composition than the traditional standard (mother, father, and children) and is indicative of twentieth-century families (single-parent, blended family, same-sex oriented couples). Domestic violence is exclusive to neither married nor heterosexual couples (Island & Letellier, 1991; Lobel, 1986; Renzetti, 1992).

The author agrees with Jones (1994) that the term "domestic violence ... [is] a euphemistic abstraction that keeps us at a dispassionate distance, far removed from the repugnant spectacle of a human being in pain" (p. 81) and prefers the term *partner abuse*. However, to stay within the limits of this chapter and maintain common terminology, *domestic violence* will refer to violence between a man and woman who are involved in an intimate relationship, with the man being the perpetrator and the woman being the victim. Between heterosexual couples, 95% of reported cases involve this dynamic (Schornstein, 1997).

Historical Perspective

Society's acceptance of violence by a man to a woman (traditionally legally united as husband and wife) originated in ancient history when "no self-respecting man would have allowed his wife to speak out against him without bashing her teeth in with a brick" (Schornstein, 1997, p. 15). During the nineteenth century judicial opinions, reflecting societal values and norms, demonstrated the callous indifference to battered women when the state supreme courts held that a husband could not be convicted of battery on his wife unless he inflicted permanent injury. The courts refused to hold a husband criminally responsible for having beaten his wife with a stick smaller than the diameter of his thumb, thus the origination of the phrase *rule of thumb*. The court held, "It is better to draw the curtain, shut out the public gaze, and leave parties to forget and forgive" (Schornstein, p. 20).

The political movement against domestic violence started by "women helping women" when, in 1848, the Seneca Falls Convention (New York) introduced the feminist movement into the United States (Jones, 1994). Yet, not until over 120 years later, in the 1970s, did the National Organization of Women make battered women a priority issue. During this same decade the first shelter for battered women was finally opened.

During the 1980s, domestic violence was recognized by governmental entities. The U.S. Commission on Civil Rights reported that at every stage of the criminal justice system victims of abuse are turned away. During this same decade mandatory arrest laws began to be passed enabling police officers to arrest perpetrators of domestic violence without having to personally witness the act. In 1994, Congress passed the Violent Crime Control and Enforcement Act, which included the Violence Against Women Act (VAWA). For the first time in the history of this country, a federal law stated domestic violence is a crime.

Strides have been made to help battered women, but they must be kept in perspective. Stated Sara Buel, assistant district attorney in Quincy, Massachusetts (and a survivor of domestic violence): "There are 1,200 shelters for battered women and their children. There are 3,900 animal protection shelters. . . . The Franklin Park Zoo got $100 million for a tropical rain forest pavilion. That same year, funding for battered women's shelters in the state was cut from $5.4 million to $4.3 million" (cited in English, 1992, p. 5).

Women Who Are Battered

"A battered woman is a woman who is repeatedly subjected to any forceful physical or psychological behavior by a man in order to coerce her to do something he wants her to do without any concern for her rights" (Walker, 1979, p. xv). Although domestic violence has no economic, religious, or racial dimensions, women who are abused share some common characteristics: low self-esteem, belief in myths of abuse (she deserved it; she is codependent), traditionalism about home, acceptance of responsibility for batterer's actions, suffering from guilt yet denying the terror and anger she feels, presentation of a passive face to the world, severe stress reactions with psychophysiological complaints, using sex as a way to establish intimacy, and belief that no one will be able to help her resolve her predicament (Walker).

Women who are in abusive relationships share similar backgrounds and consequences (NCHDBW, 1994; Walker, 1979). "As many as 80% of the women in shelters recall witnessing their mother being assaulted by their father as well as being assaulted themselves" (NCHDBW, p. 122). Approximately 50% of all female alcoholism may be precipitated by abuse. Battering may account for 25% of women who attempt suicide and 25% of women seeking emergency psychiatric care (NCHDBW). "This, then, is what battered women are for, like prostitutes (who commonly are battered women themselves), battered women serve to drain away excessive male violence and assaultive sexuality'' (Jones, 1994, p. 208).

The Batterer and Children Who Witness Domestic Violence

Batterers come from all socioeconomic backgrounds, races, religions, and occupations. While there is no typical batterer, some common behaviors do exist. Batterers are extremely manipulative and charming, maintaining a public image as a friendly, caring person who is a devoted family man. Most batterers minimize the seriousness of the violence or blame it on the victim's provocation, hold traditional views of sex roles and parenting, have negative attitudes toward women, have a history of abuse as children, are problem drinkers, and are poor problem solvers (Else et al., Wonderlich, Beatty, Christie, & Staton, 1993; Jasinski et al., 1997; NCHDBW, 1994).

Domestic violence damages the health status of every member of the family. ''Until recently the issue of child witnesses to domestic violence has occupied relatively little attention from the domestic violence research community'' (Gleason, 1995, p. 153). ''A growing body of research . . . suggests that spouse abuse and child abuse are clearly linked within families, with each being a fairly strong predictor of the other'' (McKay, 1994, p. 29). Children living in homes where domestic violence occurs suffer by becoming victims of abuse and/or witnessing the abuse (Gleason; Lehmann & Carlson, 1998; Martin, 1976; McKay; Ragg & Webb, 1992; Schornstein, 1997; Silvern & Kaersvang, 1989; Tutty & Wagar, 1994). ''Children are more than just bystanders to spousal violence'' (Gleason, p. 8).

Annually, approximately 3.3 million children witness domestic violence (NCHDBW, 1994). According to the American Medical Association (AMA), witnessing domestic violence during childhood may cause children to have a variety of physical and emotional problems that can include headaches, abdominal pain, stuttering, enuresis, and insomnia. They also demonstrate anxiety, inability to concentrate on their schoolwork, aggressive behavior, and guilt about their inability to stop the violence (Schornstein, 1997). ''Thus, in general, observing violence between parents has been found to be associated with diminished well-being in children and adolescents'' (Lehmann & Carlson, 1998, p. 101).

These adverse effects are long lasting. Adolescent boys exposed to domestic violence may use aggression as a predominant form of problem solving and have a 1,000% greater battering rate than those who have not witnessed domestic violence. Children witnessing domestic violence are six times more likely to attempt suicide, 74% more likely to commit crimes against persons, 24 times more likely to commit sexual assault crimes, and 50% more likely to abuse drugs and/or alcohol. Of imprisoned youngsters, 63% between the ages of 11 and 20 are doing time for killing their mother's batterer (NCHDBW, 1994).

Domestic violence service providers must help women recognize how their children are adversely affected by violence and must help women place responsibility for violence with the abuser (McKay, 1994). If not for their own protection, women may take action to protect their children from violence in their homes.

Dynamic of Domestic Violence

Four dynamics invariably associated with domestic violence are the Power and Control Wheel, the Cycle of Violence, Learned Helplessness, and the Battered Woman Syndrome. The Power and Control Wheel originated from The Domestic Abuse Intervention Project of Duluth, Minnesota. The tools of power and control include physical, sexual, and emotional intimidation used by the perpetrator to control his victim (Schornstein, 1997).

The Cycle of Violence, first identified by Lenore E. A. Walker (1979), includes three phases of abusive behavior. During the first phase of tension building, the victim intuitively knows the perpetrator is increasing his steps of behavior toward the abuse. The second and shortest of this circular pattern is the battering incident, when the perpetrator acts out the abuse. Following the incident, the perpetrator enters a stage of loving contrition, promising never to repeat his action and often sealing his promise with gifts. The smaller the cycle becomes, the more often and severe the battering occurs.

Learned Helplessness, as a behavior for victims of domestic violence, was extrapolated by Walker (1979) from Martin Seligman's experiment with dogs. The victim's cognitive set is systematically altered to have her believe she can no longer control what happens to her. Neither her personal worth, survival, nor autonomy depends on her responses to life situations. She is, in fact, helpless to control circumstances in her life, including her abuse by the perpetrator. More recently, literature has taken exception to this term in efforts to empower women with the ability to help themselves change their situation (Neidig, Friedman, & Collins, 1985).

The Battered Woman Syndrome (Walker, 1984) explicates the study, theories, and findings resulting in this highly debated, legal analysis of women living in abusive relationships. Battered women can be identified by their being unable to escape the cycle of violence and demonstrating the susceptibility factors for violence and learned helplessness. Among empirical findings was that "the best prediction of future violence was a history of past violence behavior" (p. 10).

Considering the abuse these women experience, the reverberating question is "Why don't they leave?" Although the answers ostensibly are relatively simplistic, the intrapsychic and societal forces precluding a battered woman's leaving are complex and perplexing. Reasons include

> economic dependence, "no place else to go," and "lacks self-confidence," . . . loving the man, believing that children need their father, hoping the marriage will improve and feeling sorry for the man. . . . Her value system can be summed up as follows: a strong belief in the institution of marriage, a desire not to harm the husband's career, a desire to avoid the embarrassment of admitting to physical and sexual abuse, a feeling of helplessness . . . [and] a feeling she is . . . responsible for the abuse. (NCHDBW, 1994, pp. 187–188)

"Women are most likely to be murdered when attempting to report abuse or to leave an abusive relationship" (NCHDBW, 1994, pp. 186–187). It is at this point when the batterer feels most threatened and vulnerable; his need to control explodes in desperate behavior. Many women go back to their batterers to stay alive (Jones, 1994).

Legal Responses

If the study of the FBI Uniform Crime Reports from 16,000 law enforcement agencies across the country were considered to be valid, domestic violence does not even exist (Jones, 1994). In the past, law enforcement often assigned low priority to domestic violence calls. When arriving at the scene, the traditional police response was merely to restore order (NCHDBW, 1994). The movie *A Cry for Help: The Tracey Thurman Story* depicts the events leading to the court's award of $2.3 million in compensatory damages by the City of Torrington, Connecticut, to

Thurman for lack of reasonable protection. The results of her suit served as a message to law enforcement officials throughout the United States to reconsider their responses to domestic violence calls (Jones).

"To be effective, any criminal justice program must begin with a policy of arresting offenders and handing out serious consequences. . . . Police must recognize assault as assault, a crime committed by a perpetrator against a victim" (Jones, 1994, p. 215). Mandatory arrest policies have been passed by an increasing number of states to provide temporary safety for victims, during which time they may seek a "Petition for Order of Protection" through the court. The judge can issue an order of "Ex Parte," a temporary restraining order, followed by a Full Order of Protection (*Domestic Violence and the Law*, nd). These policies are intended to provide safety for victims from their abusers.

The effectiveness of these policies remains unresolved and contentious. The conclusions of the Minneapolis experiment support arrests as producing the lowest percentage of repeated violence as compared with other alternatives (Witwer & Crawford, 1995). Contrary to this finding, "Sherman concludes that arrests can lead men to beat their wives and lovers more often after they are released" (NCHDBW, 1994, p. 207). "Of the 17 women killed in MA in the first eight months of 1992, 10 of them had protective orders out against their murderers" (NCHDBW, p. 200). "Women get the message that the law will not make them safe. The system does not protect them from assault at home, and it does not protect them when they leave" (Jones, 1994, p. 46).

The Role of Health Care Providers

Health care providers have enormous potential to identify and assist battered women; however, their failure to assess systematically the extent of domestic violence is well documented (Campbell, 1991; Schornstein, 1997). Each year, more than one million women seek medical treatment for injuries deliberately inflicted upon them by their husbands or boyfriends, yet doctors correctly identify these injuries in only 6% to 8% of the cases (NCHDBW, 1994; Schornstein). Their failure to talk with women about violence is attributed to opening a Pandora's box: concerns about offending patients and lack of time. By ignoring the abuse, health care providers escalate victims' entrapment and place them in increased danger by minimizing the abuse, blaming the victim, failing to respect autonomy, ignoring the need for safety, and treating the incidence as a normal occurrence (Schornstein, p. 71).

Former Surgeon General C. Everett Koop identified violence against women by their partners as the most serious health risk for women in the United States. A National Crime Survey in 1981 estimated that medical expenses arising from domestic violence were more than $44 million per year, accounting for 21,000 hospitalizations with 99,800 patient days, 28,700 emergency department visits, and 39,900 visits to physicians. This country spends $5 to $10 billion per year on health care, criminal justice, and other social service costs of domestic violence. Businesses lose $100 million annually in lost wages, sick leave, absenteeism, and nonproductivity (Schornstein, 1994). Until health care providers are willing to cooperate in a coordinated effort to identify domestic violence, millions of women and children will continue to suffer at the hands of their abusers.

Intervention Strategies for the Family Experiencing Domestic Violence

''Until now, the treatment of spouse abuse has been primarily directed at insuring that police and legal actions are available to intercede during violent episodes and at providing shelter for women who are seeking refuge from their partners'' (Neidig et al., 1985, p. 195). More recently, recognition has been given to the need for each member of the family to receive professional treatment to overcome the orientations toward violence and heal from the emotional wounds of violence (Davis & Srinivasan, 1995; McKay, 1994; O'Leary, Vivian, & Malone, 1992).

Programs for children witnessing domestic violence remain in a developmental phase relative to the need. Programs are needed in shelters for battered women and within the community. In a nationwide study of shelters for battered women, 20.3% reported ''they provide hardly any services to the children of battered women'' (Roberts, 1998, p. 68). Various models are available for children in shelters utilizing, among other strategies, short-term treatment and cognitive behavioral strategies (Alessi & Hearn, 1998; Lehmann & Carlson, 1998; O'Keefe & Lebovics, 1998). Programs for children tend to utilize group treatment (Alessi & Hearn; Pottle & Pottle, 1998; Ragg & Webb, 1992; Tutty & Wagar, 1994). During a series of structured sessions children learn social skills, problem solving, conflict resolution, and protection. Strategies include play therapy, projective drawing, story telling, and sharing of feelings. Evaluation of programs for children witnessing domestic violence is recommended to assure effectiveness of these services in breaking the chain of domestic violence.

For batterers, "the prevailing treatment approaches . . . include feminist, cognitive-behavioral, family systems, and integrative approaches. . . . Group interventions seem to work more effectively than does individual counseling" (Sakai, 1991, pp. 536, 537). The abuser must acknowledge his abusive behavior, realizing it is a choice and that he can make other, healthier choices (Caplan & Thomas, 1995; Faulkner, Cogan, Nolder, & Shooter, 1991; McKay, 1994; Sakai). Men entering a treatment group view it as punishment and a threat to their masculinity and self-worth. Provisions need to be made for the men's safety and comfort while providing the necessary content (Caplan & Thomas).

"An increasing number of models are becoming available for the treatment of couples who wish to stay together and attempt to control their violent relationship" (Neidig et al., 1985, p. 195). Break the Chain and The Domestic Conflict Containment Program are two programs developed for couples who chose to remain together. Basic principles of these programs are elimination of violence in the home, acceptance of abusiveness as a learned behavior, and violence as ineffective in the long run (Neidig et al.; A. Pottle & B. Pottle, personal communication, February 2, 1998).

Community Intervention

The Coordinated Approach to Reducing Family Violence Conference brought together over 400 professionals to foster a collaborative approach to family violence. Ten work groups submitted recommendations (Witwer & Crawford, 1995). For assessment of domestic violence, recommendations were to develop an effective, multidisciplinary, communitywide assessment process that maximizes safety for all family members and all communities to:

1. Form multidisciplinary family violence coordinating councils.
2. Develop and distribute an interdisciplinary glossary of terms and resources.
3. Establish standards for minimum community resources necessary to ensure the safety of all family members.

4. Develop community intervention referrals.
5. Evaluate effectiveness of the assessment process.
6. Develop a mechanism for the confidential sharing of appropriate information between and within various systems.

Recommendations for interventions of abuse were that all communities must (a) protect and support victims, (b) empower victims to protect themselves, (c) hold offenders accountable for past and future behavior, and (d) demand that abusers change their behaviors. To accomplish these recommendations each community should create a family violence coordinating council; the AMA should assume a major leadership role in identifying, pursuing, and obtaining long-term funding for interventions; a family violence advocate/specialist is needed in all practice settings; and a comprehensive management information system is needed to identify, evaluate, and replicate existing model family violence intervention programs. Recommendations for media were to establish a national coalition of professional organizations to work in partnership with the media to examine violence and promote socially responsible approaches.

Recommendations for prevention were (a) viewing social justice dealing with family violence in terms of affirming human rights; (b) shifting social, economic, and political resources toward strengthening communities and families, including access to employment, education, housing, and health care; (c) implementing human and financial resources at the federal, state, and local levels; and (d) integrating and sharing information among health, justice, social service, and educational systems.

Partner Violence: A 20-Year Review and Synthesis (Jasinski et al., 1997) presents a comprehensive examination of the current knowledge reflected in the literature on partner violence, with particular attention to theoretical and conceptual issues; research methods, measures, and findings; implications for policy and practice; and types and effects of interventions. This review indicates that prevention and intervention are both growing areas in the field of partner violence, with an increased focus on protective factors (e.g., problem-solving skills and strong domestic violence laws) and risk factors (e.g., alcohol abuse and community indifference). The review concludes, "There is no one solution to the problem of partner violence" (p. 10).

According to the Honorable Donna Shalala, secretary of Health and Human Services, "Family violence has become as American as guns on our streets and murders in our movies. . . . Until now, domestic violence was something the Federal Government didn't bring up. . . . We have moved from an era of closing our eyes and denying our problems to doing the tough, hard work of saving families to save futures'' (cited in Witwer & Crawford, 1995, p. ii).

Effective prevention and intervention is consistent with the family health perspective, which views the family as ''the fundamental or primary unit of a society'' whose ''functions contribute to the health and stability of society and its members'' (Pardeck, Yuen, Daley, & Hawkins, 1998, p. 28). Clearly, breaking the cycle of family violence requires participation by each and every American. As long as family violence is considered safe within the sanctity of intimate commitment and child bearing, families will be the killing fields for the American society.

REFERENCES

Alessi, J. J., & Hearn, K. (1998). Group treatment of children in shelters for battered women. In A. R. Roberts (Ed.), *Battered women and their families* (2nd ed., pp. 3–28). New York: Springer.

Ashford, J. B. (1994). Child maltreatment interventions: Developments in law, prevention, and treatment. *Criminal Justice Review, 19*(2), 271–285.

Barnett, O. W., Miller-Perrin, C. L., & Perrin, R. D. (1997). *Family violence across the lifespan: An introduction.* Thousand Oaks, CA: Sage.

Blythe, B. J. (1983). A critique of outcome evaluation in child abuse treatment. *Child Welfare League of America, 62*(4), 325–335.

Campbell, J. C. (1991). Public-health conceptions of family abuse. In D. D. Knudsen & J. L. Miller (Eds.), *Abused and battered: Social and legal responses to family violence* (pp. 49–61). New York: Aldine De Gruyter.

Caplan, T., & Thomas, H. (1995). Safety and comfort, content and process: Facilitating open group work with men who batter. *Social Work with Groups, 18*(2/3), 33–51.

Cheung, K. M., Stevenson, K. M., & Leung, P. (1991). Competency-based evaluation of case-management skills in child sexual abuse intervention. *Child Welfare League of America, 70*(4), 425–435.

Child Abuse and Neglect Laws: Related Missouri Laws. (1996). *Chapter 210, RSMO* (L. 1995 H.B. 232 & 485 and S.B. 174). 1–41. (Available through Division of Family Services, Springfield, MO, 65804).

Cohn, B. (1992, September 21). From chattel to full citizens. *Newsweek*, pp. 88–89.

Damon, L., Todd, J., & MacFarlane, K. (1987). Treatment issues with sexually abused children. *Child Welfare League of America, 66*(2), 125–137.

Davis, L. V., & Srinivasan, M. (1995). Listening to the voices of battered women: What helps them escape violence. *Affilia, 19*(1), 49–69.

Dhooper, S. S., & Schneider, P. L. (1995). Evaluation of a school-based child abuse prevention program. *Social Work Practice, 5*(1), 36–46.

Domestic violence and the law: A practical guide for survivors. (nd). The young lawyers section of the Missouri bar. (Available through Family Violence Center, P.O. Box 5972, Springfield, MO, 65801).

Else, L., Wonderlich, S. A., Beatty, W. W., Christie, D. W., & Staton, R. D. (1993). Personality characteristics of men who physically abuse women. *Hospital and Community Psychiatry, 44*(1), 54–58.

English, B. (1992, June 2). Domestic war victimizes women and children. *The Tampa Tribune*, Plant City Edition, p. 5.

Faulkner, K. K., Cogan, R., Nolder, M., & Shooter, G. (1991). Characteristics of men and women completing cognitive/behavioral spouse abuse treatment. *Journal of Family Violence, 6*(3), 243–254.

Gibbs, N. (1994, November 14). Death and deceit. *Time*, pp. 43–59.

Gleason, W. J. (1995). Children of battered women: Developmental delays and behavioral dysfunction. *Violence and Victims, 10*(2), 153–160.

Grubbs, G. A. (1994). An abused child's use of sandplaying the healing process. *Clinical Social Work Journal, 22*(2), 193–209.

Hay, T., & Jones, L. (1994). Societal interventions to prevent child abuse and neglect. *Child Welfare League of America, 83*(5), 379–403.

Helfer, R. E. (1991). Child abuse and neglect: Assessment, treatment, and prevention, October 21, 2007. *Child Abuse & Neglect, 15*(1), 5–15.

Hiebert-Murphy, D., De Luca, R. V., & Runtz, M. (1992, April). Group treatment for sexually abused girls: Evaluating outcome. *Families in Society: The Journal of Contemporary Human Services*, pp. 205–213.

Himelein, M. J., & McElrath, J. V. (1996). Resilient child sexual abuse survivors: Cognitive coping and illusion. *Child Abuse & Neglect, 20*(8), 747–758.

Island, D., & Letellier, P. (1991). *Men who beat the men who love them: Battered gay men and domestic violence*. New York: Haworth Press.

Jasinski, J. L., Williams, L. M., & Brewster, A. (1997, August 10). *Partner violence: A 20-year review and synthesis: Executive summary*. http://www.agnr.umd.edu/users/nnfr/research/pv_execsumm.html.

Jones, A. (1994). *Next time, she'll be dead: Battering & how to stop it*. Boston, MA: Beacon Press.

Kivel, P. (1992). *Unlearning violence: A breakthrough book for violent men and all those who love them*. New York: MJF Books.

Knittle, B. J., & Tuana, S. J. (1980). Group therapy as primary treatment for adolescent victims of intrafamilial sexual abuse. *Clinical Social Work Journal, 8*(4), 236–242.

Kolko, D. J. (1996). Clinical monitoring of treatment course in child physical abuse: Psychometric characteristics and treatment comparisons. *Child Abuse & Neglect, 20*(1), 23–43.

Lamb, S. (1986). Treating sexually abused children: Issues of blame and responsibility. *American Orthopsychiatric Association, 56*(2), 303–307.

Lehmann, P., & Carlson, B. E. (1998). Crisis intervention with traumatized child witnesses in shelters for battered women. In A. R. Roberts (Ed.), *Battered women and their families* (2nd ed., pp. 99–128). New York: Springer.

Lobel, K. (1986). *Naming the violence: Speaking out about lesbian battering.* Seattle, WA: National Coalition Against Domestic Violence.

McKay, M. M. (1994). The link between domestic violence and child abuse: Assessment and treatment considerations. *Child Welfare League of America, 73*(1), 29–39.

Martin, D. (1976). *Battered wives.* New York: Pocket Books.

Miller, T. W., Veltkamp, L. J., & Janson, D. (1987). Assessment of sexual abuse and trauma: Clinical measures. *Child Psychiatry and Human Development, 26*(1), 3–10.

National Clearinghouse for the Defense of Battered Women [NCHDBW]. (1994, February). *Statistics packet* (3rd ed.). Philadelphia: Author.

National Victim Center. (1995). *A decade of services.* New York: Author.

Neidig, P. H., Friedman, D. H., & Collins, B. S. (1985, April). Domestic conflict containment: A spouse abuse treatment program. *Social Casework: The Journal of Contemporary Social Work,* pp. 195–204.

Nelson, C., Miner, M., Marques, J., Russell, K., & Achterkirchen, J. (1989). *Relapse prevention: A cognitive-behavioral model for treatment of the rapist and child molester. Treatment of sex offenders in social work and mental health settings.* New York: Haworth Press.

O'Keefe, M., & Lebovics, S. (1998). Intervention and treatment strategies with adolescents from maritally violent homes. In A. R. Roberts (Ed.), *Battered women and their families* (2nd. ed., pp. 174–202). New York: Springer.

O'Leary, K. D., Vivian, D., & Malone, J. (1992). Assessment of physical aggression against women in marriage: The need for multimodal assessment. *Behavioral Assessment, 14*, 5–14.

Orten, J. D., & Rich, L. L. (1988, December). A model for assessment of incestuous families. *Social Casework: The Journal of Contemporary Social Work,* 69, pp. 611–619.

Pardeck, J. T., & Yuen, F. K. O. (1997). A family health approach to social work practice. *Family Therapy, 24*(2), 115–128.

Pardeck, J. T., Yuen, F. K. O., Daley, B., & Hawkins, K. (1998). Social work assessment and intervention through family health practice. *Family Therapy, 1*(25), 25–39.

Pottle, A., & Pottle, B. (1998). *The alternatives project. Break the chain: A program for batterers and their families.* (Available from Break The

Chain, Inc., 1031 E. Battlefield Rd., Suite 211-A, Springfield, MO, 65807).

Powell, M. P., & Wagner, W. G. (1991). Psychological evaluation of sexually abused children. *Journal of Mental Health Counseling, 13*(4), 473–485.

Ragg, D. M., & Webb, C. (1992). Group treatment for the preschool child witness of spouse abuse. *Journal of Child and Youth Care, 7*(1), 1–19.

Renzetti, C. M. (1992). *Violent betrayal: Partner abuse in lesbian relationships*. Newbury Park, CA: Sage.

Roberts, A. R. (1998). The organizational structure and function of shelters for battered women and their children: A national survey. In A. R. Roberts (Ed.), *Battered women and their families* (2nd ed., pp. 58–75). New York: Springer.

Sakai, C. E. (1991). Group intervention strategies with domestic abusers. *Families in Society: The Journal of Contemporary Human Services, 72*(9), 536–542.

Sanders, B., & Becker-Lausen, E. (1995). The measurement of psychological maltreatment: Early data on the child abuse and trauma scale. *Child Abuse & Neglect, 19*(3), 315–323.

Schornstein, S. L. (1997). *Domestic violence and health care: What every professional needs to know*. Thousand Oaks, CA: Sage.

Shorkey, C. T. (1979, June). A review of methods used in the treatment of abusing parents. *Social Casework: The Journal of Contemporary Social Work, 60*, 360–367.

Silvern, L., & Kaersvang, L. (1989). The traumatized children of violent marriages. *Child Welfare, 68*(4), 421–436.

Sink, F. (1988). A hierarchical model for evaluation of child sexual abuse. *American Orthopsychiatric Association, 58*(1), 129–135.

Tutty, L. M., & Wagar, J. (1994). The evolution of a group for young children who have witnessed family violence. *Social Work with Groups, 17*(1/2), 89–103.

Wade, S. (1997, June 26). Easy does it: Babies need tlc. *The Newsleader*, pp. 1A, 10A.

Walker, L. E. (1979). *The battered woman*. New York: Harper & Row.

Walker, L. E. (1984). *The battered woman syndrome*. New York: Springer.

Wallace, H. (1996). *Family violence: Legal, medical, and social perspectives*. Needham Heights, MA: Allyn and Bacon.

Waterman, J., & Lusk, R. (1993). Psychological testing in evaluation of child sexual abuse. *Child Abuse & Neglect, 17*, 145–159.

Winton, M. A. (1990). An evaluation of a support group for parents who have a sexually abused child. *Child Abuse & Neglect, 14*, 397–405.

Witwer, M. B., & Crawford, C. A. (1995, October). *A coordinated approach to reducing family violence: Conference highlights*. Washington, DC: U.S. Department of Justice.

Wolfner, G. D., & Gelles, R. J. (1993). A profile of violence toward children: A national study. *Child Abuse & Neglect*, *17*, 197–212.

9

An Analysis of Family Health and Family Policy

John T. Pardeck

The United States is one of the few economically developed countries that does not have an explicit national family policy. Even though the United States is one of the wealthiest countries in the world, it continues to have one of the highest rates of poverty among its citizens. Poverty among children is one of many problems facing families; other issues and social problems facing families include the following:

1. In 1960 children accounted for 36% of all Americans; in 1990 they were 26%, and by 2010 only 23% of the population will be children (U.S. Department of Commerce, Bureau of the Census, 1989b).
2. Over the past 20 years, a rapidly rising divorce rate and an increase in out-of-wedlock childbearing, particularly among teenagers, have dramatically increased the numbers of children living with one parent (U.S. Department of Commerce, 1989a).
3. One of the most dramatic changes over the past two decades has been the increasing numbers of mothers entering the work-force. Between 1970 and 1990, the proportion of mothers with children under age six who were working or looking for work

Table 9.1
Income Distribution of American Families in 1988

Population Category	Percentage of Total National Income Received	
Poorest fifth	4.6	Lowest since 1954
Second poorest fifth	10.7	Lowest ever recorded
Middle fifth	16.7	Lowest ever recorded
Richest fifth	44.0	Highest ever recorded
Richest five percent	17.2	Highest since 1952
Middle three-fifths	51.4	Lowest ever recorded

Source: O'Hare, Mann, Porter, and Greenstein (1990).

rose from 32% to 58%. In 1990, over 74% of women with children between the ages of 6 and 13 were working or looking for work (U.S. Department of Commerce, 1990).

4. Children today are the poorest Americans; one in five lives in a family below the poverty level (Cherlin, 1988).
5. Thirty-two million Americans, including 8.3 million children under age 18, have no form of health insurance coverage (National Commission on Children, 1991).
6. One in four adolescents experiences some form of serious, long-term problem (Carnegie Council on Adolescent Development, 1989). For example, approximately 1 million teenage girls become pregnant each year; half of them give birth.
7. Approximately 500,000 young people drop out of school each year (Kaufman & Frase, 1990).
8. Since 1981, there has been an 80% rise in the proportion of children receiving psychological assistance annually (Zill & Schoenborn, 1990).

One of the core factors that contributes to many problems facing families in the United States is poverty. Table 9.1 illustrates the uneven distribution of wealth of families. It can be observed in table 9.1 that the second poorest and the poorest two fifths of families receive only 15% of the nation's total income. The richest 5% receive over 17% of total income; the richest fifth receives 44%. As a result of Ronald Reagan's economic policies in the 1980s, the richest 5% of families had the greatest amount of income since 1952; the poorest fifth had the least amount since 1954. In essence, Reagan's economic strategy appeared to be to shift wealth from poor families to wealthy families. A sound family policy would do the reverse.

Given the high rates of poverty among millions of American families and the countless other social problems facing families, a reasonable conclusion can be made that children and families are under pressure in the United States. These pressures suggest that families are in need of help from the larger American society.

THE DEVELOPMENT OF AN IMPLICIT FAMILY POLICY

Even though the United States does not have an explicit comprehensive family policy, numerous programs have been developed and implemented that affect the health and well-being of families. A number of these programs were created in the mid 1930s in response to the Great Depression. Others have been created as a reaction to the various social crises since the depression. There is no grand design to these programs; they have a tendency to emphasize economic supports and are typically aimed at individuals within the family unit (Pardeck, 1990).

One of the most popular and best-known programs affecting families is the Old Age, Survivors, Disability, and Health Insurance (OASDHI), often referred to as Social Security. This program provides benefits to insured workers when they reach retirement age or become disabled. This program also provides economic support to a worker's spouse and dependent children if the insured worker dies. It is not, however, a program specifically designed to support families; it is aimed at individuals within the family system.

Public assistance is another form of economic support that has an impact on economically depressed families. The Food Stamp program and Temporary Aid to Needy Families (TANF) are examples of public assistance. Both programs require clients to meet a means test to qualify for benefits. The benefit levels for both programs are very low, and the TANF program varies dramatically in payment levels from state to state. The Food Stamp program is aimed at individuals within household units;

even though the TANF program is very new, its earlier version, entitled Aid to Families with Dependent Children (AFDC), was often found to be extremely anti-family. There is little to suggest that the TANF program will be much different from the older AFDC program.

Other examples of programs that impact the economic well-being of families are tax exemptions provided under state and federal laws and the Earned Income Tax Credit. Under the tax exemption program, families can claim family members as exemptions. Obviously, this program does not have the same effect as the children and family allowance programs found in virtually every developed country in Europe (Pardeck, 1990). The Earned Income Tax Credit (EITC) is designed for low-income families. Under this program, low-income families that have a source of income are paid a tax credit; in 1997 this tax credit was up to $2,210.

Amendments to the Social Security Act of 1935 have been aimed at improving supports and services for individuals; many of these programs have had an impact on families. For example, the 1962 and 1967 Amendments to the Social Security Act were supposed to upgrade social services to low-income children and families. As often occurs, however, the amendments were underfunded by the federal government; thus the programs added under the 1962 and 1967 Amendments had limited impact on families (Pardeck, 1990). A more recent example, the Family Welfare Act of 1988 (PL 100–485), also suffered from a lack of funding.

It is noted that there are countless services offered to children and families by nongovernmental agencies; these agencies have a tendency to serve the middle class and not poor children and their families (Pardeck, 1990). An additional criticism of these agencies is that they do not serve enough families; they simply add another layer to an already fragmented network of social services (Pardeck, 1990).

Given this situation, the following conclusions are made (Pardeck, 1990):

1. There are virtually no coordinated efforts supporting the family system through national family policy.
2. The many programs affecting families are aimed at individuals, not family units.
3. The core programs influencing family life are economic.
4. The social services offered to children and families are underfunded, uncoordinated, and limited in scope.

Critics argue that family health will only improve when the United States develops a coherent and comprehensive family policy (Pardeck, 1990). This policy should include national health care, income assistance, and comprehensive social services available to all families. A number of barriers prevent the development of this kind of national policy.

BARRIERS TO FAMILY POLICY

John T. Pardeck (1990), Robert M. Rice (1977), and Alvin L. Schorr (1972) isolated a number of factors that appear to prevent the development of a national family policy in the United States. These include:

1. A preference in the United States for limited government intervention into family life.
2. The tradition of emphasizing the individual over the family.
3. The inability to define what is meant by the family.
4. The pluralism that is characteristic of American society.

There is a clear tradition in the United States for minimal government intervention into family life. It is often feared that such intervention would be counterproductive to family well-being. One can ground this tradition in the United States Constitution, which is silent on the subject of the family. The implied contract in the Constitution is between the individual and government—this has contributed to a vacuum in the area of family policy and programs.

The pluralistic nature of American society has made it extremely difficult to reach consensus on what should be done in the way of government policy for families. Furthermore, pluralism has also made it difficult to define what is meant by the term *family*. Until these kinds of barriers are overcome, the health and well-being of families will continue to suffer (Pardeck, 1990).

EUROPEAN IDEOLOGY SUPPORTING FAMILY POLICY

Even though the United States and Europe have much in common in terms of cultural traditions, they clearly have different traditions and ideologies concerning family policy (Pardeck, 1990). John E. Tropman (1985) appears to offer an excellent explanation for why Europe and the United States differ so dramatically in the area of family policy. He argues that Europe and the United States have unique religious traditions that help to explain why one society has highly developed family policy and the other has virtually none. According to Tropman, a dominant ideology that he labels the ''catholic ethic'' is the grounding explaining why Europe has made substantial efforts aimed at supporting families. The catholic ethic finds its roots in the Roman Catholic, Anglican, and Lutheran traditions. The United States is dominated by a different religious tradition, the ''Calvinistic ethic.'' This ethic stresses the importance of the individual and self-initiative. These two religious traditions create normative standards that are markedly different in four major areas:

1. Attitudes toward poverty and social problems facing individuals and families.
2. Attitudes toward work and the meaning of work.
3. Attitudes toward charity and who should receive it.
4. The organization and structure of the welfare state.

Social Problems

The Calvinistic ethic that appears to dominate policy development in the United States views poverty as caused by laziness and lack of motivation. This tradition divides the poor into worthy and unworthy categories: The worthy are seen as those who are not responsible for being poor; such persons include people with disabilities and the elderly. The unworthy poor are those who are seen as able but simply do not want to work. Given this view, the Calvinistic tradition highly values means tests and ''safety nets'' that are temporary solutions until individuals can find work. The recent welfare reform, Personal Responsibility and Work Act of 1996 (HR 3734), includes the TANF program, a classic example of a program based on the Calvinistic ethic. Calvinism also endorses a residual approach to policy development that tends to emphasize cost cutting and is driven by crisis.

The European catholic ethic offers a much different view of needy individuals and families. This ethic has resulted in family programs grounded in the position that families have limited control over social problems and are often victims of them. Tropman (1985) even suggests that the catholic ethic views excessive wealth as spiritually dangerous. Thus the distribution of wealth to families in need is seen as a duty.

Consequently, an impulse toward mutual obligation and social welfare is stressed.

The catholic and Calvinistic ethics help to explain why Europe and the United States differ tremendously in the area of family policy. Virtually every European country has a children and family allowance; no such program exists in the United States. European countries offer health care to all citizens; approximately 32 million persons in the United States have no health insurance (Karger & Stoesz, 1994; National Commission on Children, 1991). The tax systems in Europe tend to be progressive; they are regressive in the United States. European countries are largely composed of middle-class families and poverty is nearly nonexistent, whereas in the United States millions of children and their families live below the poverty level. The Calvinistic ethic contributes to the trend of not supporting family programs; this trend means many American families will continue to lack critical social services, adequate nutrition, shelter, and health care (Pardeck, 1990).

Work

Under the Calvinistic ethic, personal worth is measured by individual productivity. The catholic ethic suggests a contrasting view that stresses the worth of the individual as determined by what he or she contributes to society; thus work has an instrumental meaning reflected in providing clothing, food, and shelter for oneself and one's family. Under the catholic ethic, work is seen as a creative process that benefits society and enhances the talents of individuals.

The Calvinistic ethic has influenced the worldview of many Americans toward work. Work defines the very essence of how one perceives the self and others; those who do not work are seen as less worthy and less important to the larger society. The Calvinistic ethic strongly suggests that welfare programs stifle the work ethic; thus it is easy for policymakers to justify not having supports and programs for families in need. Such programs would, presumably, deter individuals from working. Furthermore, a number of theorists have argued that the true function of the limited number of U.S. welfare programs is nothing more than a tool for regulating the poor (Piven & Cloward, 1971). Frances Piven and Richard Cloward argue that private industry has a vested interest in keeping welfare benefits low during times of economic prosperity in order to insure workers' choosing work over relief. Historically, a major argument against family allowances and other supports has been that such programs encourage relief over work (Pardeck, 1990).

The new welfare reform of 1996 (HR 3734) heavily emphasizes work over welfare. This "Workfare" focus has been characteristic of many welfare programs created in the United States. Clearly the Calvinistic ethic is a grounding for this tradition.

European countries have a much different view of work, one that suggests the American orientation toward work and welfare may be inaccurate. Even though Europe has highly developed family policies, there is little or no evidence to suggest that these policies stifle the work ethic (Pardeck, 1990). One might even argue that the inability of the United States to respond to oppressed families through policy and programs is creating a dangerous social class that might potentially destabilize the larger society. Presently there are nearly two million homeless families in the United States, a major social problem that must be dealt with (Karger & Stoesz, 1994). Postindustrial society demands that families must receive appropriate economic and social supports in order for the community and larger society to be healthy. Adequate health care, day care, and other family supports are a necessity in a postindustrial society.

Charity

Tropman (1985) suggests that the catholic ethic stresses a horizontal relationship between the individual and others, while the Calvinistic ethic offers a vertical view of human relationships. These views translate into different perspectives concerning the importance and meaning of community.

Tropman (1985) concludes that the catholic ethic results in a greater sense of community and commitment to one another. This ethic may explain why European countries have progressive tax systems that have created a strong middle class and virtually eliminated poverty. It also provides insight into why most European countries have children and family allowances. Such supports help the larger society realize its commitment to children and families. Such programs illustrate commitment to the importance of horizontal human relationships grounded in the catholic ethic.

Calvinism takes a dramatically different view than the catholic ethic concerning the meaning and importance of charity. Calvinism views charity as a negative that should only be provided under the most dire circumstances. Given this view, it makes perfect sense that poverty, homelessness, and other social problems are far more pronounced in the United States than in Europe. Until this worldview changes, family policy will be difficult to develop in the United States.

Organizational Structure

The final element of the catholic versus the Calvinistic ethic concerns how each views the bureaucratic structures that deliver social welfare programs. The catholic ethic endorses a positive view of the bureaucratic structure that is critical to effective social service delivery. Tropman (1985) suggests that this tradition is connected to tolerance of a highly developed church structure that has simply been replaced by a developed welfare state. The Calvinistic ethic, as would be expected, has a much different position on the organizational structures critical to the delivery of social services. The Calvinistic view is suspicious of highly developed church structures; this view carries over to welfare bureaucratic structures. Under the Calvinistic ethic, the person and his or her family is responsible for meeting needs, not the welfare state.

The origins of the catholic and Calvinistic ethics hardly defy explanation. The Calvinistic Reformation radically reduced the medieval ecclesiastical institutional structure. The church policy became congregational; the Puritan minister stood alone at the head of the local assembly. That aloneness may well have given rise to the ideal of self-reliance, not merely in the religious sphere but in life in general. The ideology of self-reliance has become a dominant theme throughout the United States and clearly has had a major impact on the family policy development (Pardeck, 1990).

A MODEL FAMILY POLICY SUPPORTING FAMILY HEALTH

A model national policy for children and their families must accommodate the pluralistic nature of American society. The policy should be built on the political, economic, and social diversity of the American population. However, it must have a degree of centralized control to insure social justice for children and their families. Given the political and economic diversity of the United States, highly centralized children and family programs as found in European countries do not serve as appropriate models for the United States (Chung & Pardeck, 1997).

Political dialogue focusing on children and family programs has been continuous for a number of decades. Regardless of the outcome of this dialogue, Sheila Kamerman and Alfred Kahn (1976) concluded over two decades ago that no developed society can avoid programs for children and their families. They suggest the real choice is between a consistent, coherent family policy and one of inconsistency and mischance. Two notable classic studies provide clear guidelines for a coherent national family policy: *Toward a National Policy for Children and Families* (National Research Council, 1976) and *All Our Children* (Keniston & The Carnegie Council on Children, 1977).

Toward a National Policy for Children and Families concludes that the federal government must take the lead in developing a comprehensive national policy for children and families; the core components of the policy should include:

1. Employment, tax, and cash benefit programs that assure each child's family an adequate income.
2. A broad and carefully integrated system of support services available to all children and their families.
3. Planned and coordinated mechanisms that ensure adequate coverage and access of families to a full range of social services and health care.

In order to implement this national policy, specific policies and programs focusing on economic resources, health care, child care, and special services need to be developed. It also recommends that research aimed at improving the knowledge base for all programs concerning America's children is a necessity.

All Our Children makes similar recommendations to those offered by *Toward a National Policy for Children and Families. All Our Children* suggests that a broad, well-integrated, explicit children and family policy should include the following:

1. Jobs should be provided for parents, and a decent living standard must be made available to all families. This would be accomplished through full employment, fair employment, and a decent minimum-income level for all.
2. There must be support in the policy for more flexible working conditions. The demands of a parent's employment should conflict as little as possible with the needs of the family.
3. The policy should have an integrated network of family services.

Federal standards for quality and fairness should be enacted for all family services.

4. The policy should include proper health care for all children as an essential goal. Recognition is needed of the fact that children's health depends as much on income, environment, and diet as it does on hospitals, nurses, and pediatricians.
5. The policy should be aimed at improving the legal protections for children outside and inside their families. The law should make every effort to keep families together.

These classic studies, *Toward a National Policy for Children and Families* and *All Our Children*, stress the importance of economic supports for families, health care for children and families, and comprehensive social services. However, *All Our Children* places greater emphasis on children's rights and also stresses the issue of flexible working hours for parents (Chung & Pardeck, 1997).

Most of the recommendations offered in *Toward a National Policy for Children and Families* and *All Our Children* are realistic programs for a national family policy. The model national policy offered below integrates several ideas from each of these studies. The core philosophy upon which the proposed model for a family policy rests is that the family is a vital social system critical to the well-being of children and the larger society. Peter L. Berger and Robert Neuhaus (1977, p. 8) describe the essence of the philosophy guiding the proposed model policy: "(It) means public recognition of the family as an institution. It is not enough to be concerned for individuals more or less incidentally related to the family as an institution. Public recognition of the family as an institution is imperative because every society has an inescapable interest in how children are raised and how values are transmitted to the next generation."

Keeping the above points in mind, the proposed model family policy includes the following (Chung & Pardeck, 1997):

1. There should be a decent standard of living for all children and families in America. This standard of living should be created through guaranteed jobs in the private sector and government. Every head of a household would be guaranteed a job. If a household head were not able to work, the family would be provided a minimum income.

2. Comprehensive health care for the entire family would be imperative. This should not be a policy only for the children of a family but for the parents as well. The policy must emphasize total health care by stressing the importance of diet, environment, and preventive health care. The policy would be designed to keep families together during a health crisis. Currently, because of exorbitant health care costs, many families experience tremendous economic pressure when a family member is sick.
3. Comprehensive social services must be offered to meet the needs of the modern family. No doubt, many of the current problems facing the family could be solved if services were available to all children and their families. The services offered would include child care, counseling services, and services for special problems, including permanent or temporary separation from the family. Comprehensive social services would be a dramatic departure from the traditional approaches to assisting the family, which are mainly in the form of economic support programs such as social insurance and public welfare.
4. The policy must provide for expanded research concerning the family. The goal of this research would be to gauge family needs. The research would emphasize three main areas: (a) studies of the family in its natural setting, (b) systematic experimentation with and evaluation of programs proposed for children and families, and (c) the development of social indicators dealing with children. The main thrust of this research would be to further the understanding of the problems of the family as a social system. As suggested by Pardeck (1990), too much current research is aimed at the individual in the family and not at the family as a social system.

In the final analysis, a comprehensive family policy must be designed to provide a decent standard of living for all families, comprehensive health care for children and their parents, quality social services, and research focused on the needs of the entire family system (Chung & Pardeck, 1997).

FAMILY HEALTH AND THE PERSONAL RESPONSIBILITY AND WORK ACT OF 1996 (HR 3734)

The Personal Responsibility and Work Act of 1996 is a dramatic departure from prior welfare policy. One of the major provisions of the new welfare reform is to move welfare policy and programs from the federal level to the state and local levels. Even though the verdict is not yet in on the new welfare reform, it does not appear to be family friendly. The major provisions of HR 3734 include the following:

1. The Aid to Families with Dependent Children (AFDC) program is replaced by the Temporary Assistance to Needy Families (TANF) program. This new program will be largely run by the states and local governments.
2. Under TANF, states receive a block grant that will be capped. States will have great discretion in how they spend the TANF money. However, once the block grant is spent, states are not entitled to additional funds. A contingency fund is established to help states which spend in excess of their block grant amounts; this funding will only be available under limited conditions, specifically during times of high unemployment.
3. Adults who receive cash benefits are required to work or participate in a state-designed work program after two years; if they do not participate, they will lose benefits. The requirement mandates that one individual in a household must work at least 30 hours a week.
4. States must have at least 50% of their total single-parent welfare cases in jobs by 2002. States that do not meet this requirement will have their block grants reduced by 5% each year until they achieve compliance.
5. States can sanction clients who fail to meet the work requirement through reduction or termination of cash benefits.
6. Payments to recipients using federal funds must end after a maximum of five years; clients must be self-supporting at that point.
7. Food Stamps are cut for individuals between the ages of 18 and 50 years.
8. Many children with disabilities will be declared ineligible for Supplemental Security Income (SSI).
9. Persons immigrating to the United States after the passage of HR 3734 are ineligible for most means-tested government programs, including TANF, Food Stamps, and Medicaid, for the first five years of residence.
10. Illegal aliens are barred from all means-tested programs.

Given the discretion that states have in implementing HR 3734, this new welfare reform will simply contribute to the further fragmentation of programs affecting family health. It creates 50 distinct and different welfare states within the United States. The real meaning of HR 3734 is that it will contribute to greater uncertainty for families and does not appear to promote family and individual well-being.

Cindy Mann (1996), in a policy analysis of the impact of HR 3734 on individuals and families in one state, Missouri, reports the following:

1. No poor child or family in Missouri will be assured of economic assistance. Temporary Assistance to Needy Families is a block grant, not a program.
2. The block grants under HR 3734 are frozen; when Missouri experiences economic downturn, only a limited amount of contingency funds will be available from the federal government.
3. The maximum time period a family can receive TANF in Missouri is five years.
4. The grant to a family of three under TANF is $292, an amount well below the poverty level.
5. Medicaid eligibility and receipt of aid under TANF are delinked. Thus many TANF families will not automatically receive Medicaid as they did under AFDC.
6. Unemployed, employable adults not raising children are limited to three months of Food Stamps in a three-year time period—24,000 people will lose Food Stamps because of this rule in the state of Missouri.
7. Legal immigrants and their families will be denied Food Stamps and SSI in Missouri. In 1999, 1,200 legal immigrants will lose their SSI support.
8. In Missouri, an estimated 7,600 children with disabilities will lose SSI.

Mann (1996) clearly illustrates that the impact of HR 3734 will be very negative for children and families in Missouri. No doubt HR 3734 will have a similar effect in other states. Thus the tradition of limited family policy continues within the United States through this new welfare reform. The result is that millions of children and families will go without adequate health care, social services, and economic supports.

REFERENCES

Berger, P. L., & Neuhaus, R. (1977). *To empower people: The role of mediating structures in public policy*. Washington, DC: American Enterprise Institute for Public Policy Research.

Carnegie Council on Adolescent Development. (1989). *Turning points: Preparing American youth for the 21st century*. Washington, DC: Author.

Cherlin, A. J. (1988). *The changing American family and public policy*. Washington, DC: Urban Institute Press.

Chung, W. S., & Pardeck, J. T. (1997). Explorations in a proposed national family policy for children and families. *Adolescence, 32*, 429–436.

Kamerman, S., & Kahn, A. (1976). Explorations in family policy. *Social Work, 21*, 181–186.

Karger, H., & Stoesz, D. (1994). *American social welfare policy: A pluralist approach* (2nd ed.). New York: Longman.

Kaufman, P., & Frase, M. J. (1990). *Dropout rates in the United States: 1989*. Washington, DC: U.S. Department of Education.

Keniston, K., & The Carnegie Council on Children. (1977). *All our children*. New York: Harcourt Brace Jovanovich.

Mann, C. (1996). *The new welfare law: The impact on the safety net*. Jefferson City, MO: Center on Budget and Policy Priorities.

National Commission on Children. (1991). *Beyond rhetoric: A new American agenda for children and families*. Washington, DC: Government Printing Office.

National Research Council. (1976). *Toward a national policy for children and families*. Washington, DC: National Academy of Sciences.

O'Hare, W., Mann, T., Porter, K., & Greenstein, R. (1990). *Real life poverty in America: Where the American public would set the poverty line*. Washington, DC: Population Reference Bureau, Inc. and the Center on Budget and Policy Priorities.

Pardeck, J. T. (1990). An analysis of the deep social structure preventing the development of a national policy for children and families in the United States. *Early Child Development and Care, 57*, 23–30.

Piven, F., & Cloward, R. (1971). *Regulating the poor: The functions of public welfare*. New York: Random House.

Rice, R. M. (1977). *American family policy: Content and context*. New York: Family Service Association of America.

Schorr, A. L. (1972). *Exploration in social policy*. New York: Basic Books.

Tropman, J. E. (1985). The "Catholic ethic" vs. the Protestant ethic: Catholic social services and the welfare state. *Social Thought, 12*, 13–22.

U.S. Department of Commerce, Bureau of the Census. (1989a). *Projections of the population of the United States No. 1018: Projections of the population in the United States by age, sex, and race*. Washington, DC: Government Printing Office.

U.S. Department of Commerce, Bureau of the Census. (1989b). *Projections of the population of the United States No. 168: Money income and poverty status in the United States*. Washington, DC: Government Printing Office.

U.S. Department of Commerce, Bureau of the Census. (1990). *Current population reports No. 447: Household and family characteristics*. Washington, DC: Government Printing Office.

Zill, N., & Schoenborn, C. A. (1990). *Developmental, learning and emotional problems: Health of our nation's children, United States, 1988*. Hyattsville, MD: U.S. Department of Health and Human Services, National Center for Health Statistics.

10

Postmodernism, Family Health, and Reflexivity in Social Work Practice

John T. Murphy, John T. Pardeck, and Karen A. Callaghan

TRADITIONAL SCIENCE

Social work is a discipline that is trying to become knowledge based. In the not so distant past, social workers based their interventions on intuition, empathy, and personal experience. Nowadays, however, these criteria are considered to be entirely too soft and imprecise. Professional social work requires that rigorous and reliable standards be employed to design, implement, and evaluate interventions.

As a result of this belief, knowledge-based interventions have become synonymous with the use of science. Accordingly, the course work in social work programs has been upgraded to include training in research techniques, statistics, and computer applications. Decision making, moreover, is thought to be aided greatly by the widespread introduction of a host of standardized tests and clinical indices. And in some cases, interventions are selected by expert systems. In the end, clinical experience and empathy are overshadowed by a myriad of techniques and instruments (Murphy & Pardeck, 1991).

This shift in priorities is thought to enhance the objectivity of clinical decision making and the accuracy of interventions. But why is so much faith placed in science? Why is clinical intervention assumed to be improved simply because it is predicated on science?

In a very traditional manner, practitioners have succumbed to the claims made about science. Specifically, they have accepted the usual proposals that science is value free and unbiased. And with personal idiosyncrasies systematically eliminated, interventions will undoubtedly be improved. Science, in short, represents a style of investigation that is qualitatively different from any other kind; science is disinterested and unaffected by the contingencies associated with the human element (Longino & Murphy, 1995).

Value neutrality can be associated with science because of a specific, and questionable, theoretical demarche. In short, traditional science is underpinned by Cartesian dualism. What René Descartes argues is that the *res extensa* and *res cogito* can and should be kept separate. In more modern terminology, he is arguing that subjectivity and objectivity are categorically distinct, and thus objects of knowledge are not necessarily tied to human praxis, cognition, language use, or any other source of distortion. As a result of this dualism, a location is available where knowledge can reside that is uncontaminated by the human presence. Moreover, methods can be invented that provide privileged access to this realm.

Through the use of formalization, the image is created that certain procedures and practices transcend the melange of conflicting claims that comprise everyday life (Bordo, 1987). For example, methodological protocol are transformed into step-wise instructions, which do not need to be interpreted as they are implemented. As a result, these practices are not disrupted by human intentions and provide unimpaired access to facts. Indeed, scientific methodology acts simply as a conduit for information.

Using logic, algorithms, specialized scripts, and other supposedly culture-free means to summarize findings serves a similar function. Information is organized in what appears to be a mechanistic manner, divorced from interpretation and other sources of human error. Categories are available to sort information that appears to be universal, while equally unbiased and standardized procedures can be invoked to test the significance of any differences that are found. Consistent with Cartesianism, the aim of science is to escape from the influence of subjectivity and encounter brute reality. Given this promise, the lure of science has been strong among clinical practitioners.

THE LINGUISTIC TURN

The ability of science to escape from the influence of *quotidian* concerns has been thwarted lately by several theories. These approaches to theory can be placed under the general heading of postmodernism (Murphy, 1989). As might be suspected, the overall thrust of this trend is to undermine dualism. And with dualism in jeopardy, claims about value freedom, disinterestedness, and the empirical character of facts lose credibility.

These postmodern writers have taken what is called a "linguistic turn." While basing their writing on the later work of Ludwig Wittgenstein, they reject the metaphysics that is at the root of science. They abandon, in short, any pretense to encountering brute reality. As part of this shift in orientation, they contend there is no clear path, or method, that leads to this exalted res extensa. The zero point coveted by scientists does not exist; or better yet, this region is an illusion perpetrated by dualism.

Following Wittgenstein, postmodernists argue that all knowledge is mediated by language (Lyotard, 1984). What these writers are refuting is the indexical theory of language, whereby speech acts point to, indicate, or highlight important facets of the world. Presupposed by this thesis is that reality is unscathed by the linguistic pointer and provides an objective referent for language. Postmodernists disagree with this assessment because of the presence of dualism.

Central to this disagreement is their belief that nothing exceeds the influence of language. In other words, nothing escapes untouched by the influence of interpretation. For this reason, postmodernists concur with Wittgenstein that reality constitutes simply a composite of "language games" (Lyotard, 1984, pp. 9–11). Because of the confluence of language and reality, speech acts influence greatly the search for knowledge and the identity of all discoveries.

Rather than objective in the Cartesian sense, reality is found within the nuances of speech. As a result, Wittgenstein argued that philosophers were no longer necessary. After all, their usual bailiwick has disappeared—there is no longer any justification for searching for the usual absolutes. Because there is no "other side" of language, access to these universals is blocked (Barthes, 1977, p. 30). And while scientists may still be valuable, their status is also affected by this rejection of dualism.

According to postmodernists, science represents a language game. In current parlance, science emerges from a particular and unique mode of discourse (Foucault, 1989). What is thought to be an unbiased search for knowledge, therefore, is actually based on certain preconditions. Rather than a pristine vehicle for unearthing truth, scientific research is pervaded by a linguistically inscribed image of existence.

Another way of making this point is to recognize that science is an embedded phenomenon. Similar to every other aspect of social life, science has a biography that contains, among other things, an origin and a destiny that are constructed in an ongoing manner. The search for facts and all conclusions are affected appreciably by this history. In the end, science is a normative endeavor, rather than value free.

THE CULTURE OF SCIENCE

What some contemporary writers, such as Mary Hesse (1980), recognize is that science embodies a culture. This position is somewhat more radical than the one provided by Thomas S. Kuhn (1996), where science is understood to be comprised of shifting paradigms. According to this cultural scenario, for example, there is no normal science that can be contrasted to less pristine versions. Instead, all science is pervaded by particular renditions of fact, truth, causality, and so forth.

In the absence of dualism, science is connected intimately to language use. Science is thus a mode of human praxis; science represents a unique accomplishment, a particular way of engaging the world. Moreover, this type of engagement is accompanied by particular commitments, values, rules, and behavioral expectations. As Husserl (1972) argues, science is a regional ontology, otherwise known as a self-contained world.

For example, in this world facts are linked to empirical indicators; empirically verifiable properties provide the basis of facticity. In this regard, subjectivity is an impediment to reaching this source of truth. Accordingly, standardized methodologies—such as psychiatric indices or other assessment instruments—are thought to best capture these facts. In point of fact, claims that are not verified by these methods are dismissed regularly as illusory. Only so-called hard data are considered to be worthy of serious attention.

And like any other culture, science has several liabilities. First, the benefits of this culture are not immediately obvious to everyone. A long period of socialization, sometimes including graduate training, is necessary to gain entry to this culture. Second, the culture of science is not necessarily universal; disseminating this culture requires the use of sophisticated rhetoric and, sometimes, coercion. Third, science can come into conflict with other cultures, thereby suggesting the need for a reconciliation process.

What has happened in the modern world, however, is that this side of science has been overlooked. Science transcends the boundaries of culture, according to the usual bromide, and resolves conflict among less universal viewpoints. Much closer to the truth is that science imposes a particular worldview. This viewpoint, furthermore, is not thought to be mired in the problems associated with traditionally conceived cultures. In other words, providing science with such an exalted position is a variant of cultural supremacy. The culture of science is simply devoid of the flaws inherent to other cultures, and therefore all rational persons are expected to adopt this outlook to guide their search for valid knowledge.

SCIENCE AND ETHNOCENTRISM

When any perspective is presumed to be objective and neutral, many problems can arise. At first, this charge sounds counterintuitive. How can objectivity, the usual guarantor of ethical propriety, be the cause of methodological or social difficulties? The commonly held opinion is that objectivity is linked to fairness and justice; objectivity is the antidote to myopic tendencies.

Despite these views, objectivity is not innocent. Persons can be lulled into compliancy by claims of objectivity and thus fail to recognize that a perspective is always operative. In the case of science, this fear is very real. Because of the alleged universality of science, this approach to conceptualizing the world has been allowed to overwhelm all others. Little thought has been given to the idea that objective assessments can systematically mask the truth of a situation. How can objectivity possibly compromise the search for truth? Becoming increasingly scientific is almost synonymous with progress and achieving wisdom.

Nonetheless, what has occurred is that science has become ethnocentric. Consistent with a general definition of ethnocentrism, the culture of science has come into conflict regularly with other cultures. As described by Alfred Schutz (1962), the so-called higher level concepts used by scientists to describe reality have replaced the ones used by persons in everyday discourse to organize their lives. What he calls the primary existential categories have been usurped by the language game of science. The aim of this substitution, of course, is to increase rigor and objectivity. The concepts that are a part of natural language are believed to be too sloppy or fuzzy for inclusion in scientific analysis. Scientific *heuristics*—a term that has a patina of objectivity—are thus introduced to improve the quality of the information that is generated.

Although this proposal has face validity, ethnocentrism is present. Clearly, the culture of those who are studied is considered to be inferior to the culture of science. As a result, nonscientific cultures are not assessed in their own terms; these other realities are made to conform to the structures imposed by science. For example, behavior is often translated by clinical indices into syndromes that are considered to be indicative of deficiency or pathology. In practically any other circumstance not prescribed by science, reductionism such as this would be deemed unacceptable. Still, this transformation occurs almost on a daily basis among practitioners.

Without a doubt, ethnocentrism is dehumanizing, even when this form of prejudice is enacted through science. Persons are not treated as ends in themselves but are made into examples or cases. They are stripped of any ability to define themselves and their surroundings and are cataloged in ways that are culturally insensitive and harmful. The narrative that is told in a particular locale is simply obscured behind an armamentarium of methods, concepts, and rules that are thought to enhance this tale. In the end, however, this conflict between cultures is very damaging to those that are identified as nonscientific. As in every example of ethnocentrism, social possibilities are unnecessarily narrowed and distorted (Pardeck & Yuen, 1997).

FAMILY HEALTH AND REFLEXIVITY

The ethnocentrism that has become a part of traditional science is especially damaging to the family health approach to intervention. Terms such as *holistic, broad, sensitive*, and *inclusive* are associated with this strategy. Family health practitioners recognize that social problems are embedded within a host of interlocking social formations. Accordingly, interventions will likely be inappropriate unless entry is gained to these areas of social life and the complexity of a presenting problem is appreciated.

To employ a term popularized by phenomenologists, the Liebenswelt, or ''life-world,'' is understood to be the framework that defines the norms of health and illness in the family health model (Husserl, 1970). What this declaration means is that these standards are socially constructed, have local relevance, and are tied to a myriad of interpersonal considerations. Behavior, therefore, cannot be identified properly by merely consulting empirical indicators or by relying on the usual clinical indices. For in each case, the existential considerations that supply behavior with meaning can be easily overlooked.

What this type of embeddedness requires is sensitivity that is antitheoretical to the culture of science. *A prioris* standards of objectivity, in other words, block access to the interpretive regions of social life where the distinctions are enacted that determine the parameters of health and illness. As noted earlier, these aprioris narrow a practitioner's vision, although initially these ideals may be comforting. Most often, narrowness and objectivity are not linked.

Instead of value freedom, the success of the family health model is derived from the use of interventions that are value relevant. Therefore, clients should be understood in their own terms, so their cultural backgrounds become apparent. Their natural language and its various social formations should be penetrated, thus providing insight into how illness is defined, expected to occur, and treated by the members of a particular community. But knowledge such as this will not be readily forthcoming as long as practitioners continue to believe a proper intervention can be designed only according to the heuristics of science.

Value relevance in this context refers to the need to view a community through its own eyes. In this regard, priority is placed on "communicative competence" in the family health model (Habermas, 1970). Rather than coveting objectivity—distance and disinterestedness—practitioners should strive to engage clients in dialogue. Every assessment instrument that is adopted, accordingly, should be viewed as providing an opportunity for achieving intimacy. As opposed to gathering facts, practitioners should view themselves as trying to enter the world of a client.

To be effective, those who adhere to the family health model realize they must become "reflexive" when inaugurating an intervention. What is encompassed by this activity, according to writers such as Alvin Gouldner (1970) and Niklas Luhmann (1995), is the ability to review critically the various assumptions that ground different theories of behavior, clinical instruments, or other facets of the intervention process. As a result of exposing these presuppositions, their range of relevance can be explicitly noted. And once these limitations are revealed, the need to assess clients in their own terms becomes apparent. Through reflexivity, issues of relevance and proper interpretation are brought to the forefront in a manner that is not important when objectivity is stressed.

This ability to be reflexive stems from the rejection of dualism. If persons have an active mind that engages reality, this cognitive activity can interrogate itself. The role that interpretation plays in the formation of assessment protocol and clinical instruments, for example, can thus be revealed, while a determination is made about whether or not these modes of constructing social reality are situationally relevant. And as relevance is improved, understanding is likewise enhanced. As should be noted, reflexivity is significant in establishing the communicative competence required to appreciate fully the embeddedness of norms.

THE FAMILY HEALTH APPROACH AND INTERVENTION

Anyone who adopts the family health model should remember the following points:

1. Value freedom is a myth; even claims about objectivity represent a particular perspective. Because the mind is understood to be active, neutrality is not possible. Furthermore, the products of cognition, even science, are imbued with specific values, beliefs, and commitments. Clinical instruments, accordingly, construct a reality, as opposed to simply garnering facts.
2. Because of this constructivist epistemology, behavior is understood to be embedded within a range of social formations. These arrangements are symbolic—linguistic—in nature and embody norms that are engendered and supported through ongoing discourse. Therefore, conceptions of health and illness reflect the intricacies of specific social relationships and should not be presumed to be universal.
3. A successful intervention requires that behavior be understood in its own terms; behavior must not be assessed outside of the social interaction that provides it with significance. Accordingly, practitioners should recognize that clinical instruments can easily become ethnocentric as a result of requiring that behavior be operationalized according to the dictates of the culture of science. This unfortunate outcome is especially likely when practitioners are enamored of objectivity and thus avoid recognizing how standardized instruments can become reductionistic. Persons cannot be understood in their own terms when achieving

objectivity requires that natural language and any influence of interpretation be avoided.

4. According to the family health model, an intervention should be based on communicative competence. Most important is that effective communication requires that the pragmatic thrust of language be acknowledged. Clinicians, accordingly, must attempt to enter the existential world of their clients. In a manner of speaking, interventions should be built from the ground up, so that unfounded aprioris do not distort what a client is trying to express.
5. Reflexivity should be viewed as a vital component of any intervention. Nonetheless, according to traditional science, this activity is disruptive and can easily lead to error. Within the family health perspective, however, reflexivity constitutes the type of self-examination that is essential to developing a nonreductionistic intervention. Without a critical review of assumptions, cultural insensitivity is difficult to avoid.

In the end, the family health model is empowering to clients. They are given the latitude to construct themselves and their world, including any problems that may arise. Furthermore, their insights and recommendations are viewed to be vital to a successfully designed intervention. Clinical experts, in this sense, are directed by their clients to examine considerations that might otherwise remain outside of a treatment plan. In this regard, the family health model is truly client centered.

In general, the family health model is predicated on an epistemology that encourages methodological pluralism. Clients are envisioned to be implicated within a web of meanings that holds the key to assessing properly any malady. Dynamism and openness are characteristic of an intervention that is inspired by the family health model (Feyerabend, 1975). What else can be the case, when the way in which a client constructs the world specifies how an intervention should proceed?

REFERENCES

Barthes, R. (1977). *Image, music, and text.* New York: Hill and Wang.

Bordo, S. (1987). *The flight to objectivity.* Albany, NY: State University of New York Press.

Feyerabend, P. (1975). *Against method.* London: Verso.

Foucault, M. (1989). *The archaeology of knowledge*. London: Routledge.

Gouldner, A. (1970). *The coming crisis in Western sociology*. New York: Basic Books.

Habermas, J. (1970). Toward a theory of communicative competence. In H. P. Dreitzel (Ed.), *Recent sociology* (2nd ed., pp. 114–148). New York: Macmillan.

Hesse, M. (1980). *Revolutions and reconstructions in the philosophy of science*. Bloomington: Indiana University Press.

Husserl, E. (1970). *The crisis in European sciences and transcendental phenomenology*. Evanston, IL: Northwestern University Press.

Husserl, E. (1972). *Ideas*. New York: Collier-Macmillan.

Kuhn, T. S. (1996). *The structure of scientific revolutions* (3rd ed.). Chicago, IL: University of Chicago Press.

Longino, C. F., & Murphy, J. W. (1995). *The old-age challenge to the biomedical model*. Amityville, NY: Baywood.

Luhmann, N. (1995). *Social systems*. Stanford, CA: Stanford University Press.

Lyotard, J. F. (1984). *The postmodern condition*. Minneapolis: University of Minnesota Press.

Murphy, J. W. (1989). *Postmodern social analysis and criticism*. Westport, CT: Greenwood Press.

Murphy, J. W., & Pardeck, J. T. (1991). *The computerization of social service agencies: A critical appraisal*. Westport, CT: Auburn House.

Pardeck, J. T., & Yuen, F. K. O. (1997). A family health approach to social work practice. *Family Therapy*, *24*, 115–128.

Schutz, A. (1962). *Collected papers* (Vol. I). The Hague: Nijhoff.

11

Family Health–centered Community Practice

Lola M. Butler and Diane Elliott

The focus of this chapter is family health–centered practice in the community. It is the authors' view that just as "it takes a village to raise a child," it takes a community to promote family health. This chapter explores the dynamics of the community environment—its function, role, and responsibility in improving and enhancing the quality of family health. The authors address strategies and solutions that enable communities to respond effectively to family health issues.

In this chapter the authors provide expanded definitions for family, health, family health, and community. They also identify the theoretical underpinnings used to explicate the concepts presented here. The authors explore action theory from the social constructionist school as an empowering framework for intervention with the community. They describe alternative theories that are appropriate in conceptualizing and defining communities and present a historical overview of traditional communities and how they change. Finally, the authors offer potential solutions for micro-, mezzo-, and macrolevels of intervention with the community.

In recent years many health and human service professionals have been slowly coming to the conclusion that individualized approaches and interventions to social welfare issues are often lacking in scope. According to H. Hugh Floyd (1980), the family has become the focus of much concern over the past two decades as a variety of family health–related problems have become major social issues. These sociopsychological problems are considered to have negative consequences at the individual, family, and community levels.

When any of these factors are out of balance, a holistic state of well-being can be threatened. For example, one such issue is substance abuse. The far-reaching effect of this social problem has been well documented in relation to its impact on the individual, family, and society. At the individual level, substance abuse can result in a person's inability to provide for one's basic survival needs through job and income loss, not to mention the impact of the abuse on one's health. Legal ramifications can also be a consequence of this type of abuse. The fact that most individuals and families do not have the means to control the flow of illegal drugs in and outside of the country indicates that societal interventions and social policies are essential.

To address family health requires that the social structure of the community be employed to respond appropriately to a comprehensive or holistic state of family health. In other words, the community has a role in facilitating the well-being of its members. Many social systems, institutions, organizations, and individuals must be involved in the process (Daly, Jennings, Beckett, & Leashore, 1995). Nontraditional definitions of community can serve as a viable strategy.

DEFINITION OF TERMS

Family, *health*, *family health*, and *community* are terms used throughout this chapter; they are defined within the context of the discussion.

Family

A *family* is seen as a primary group whose members assume certain obligations, functions, and responsibilities for each other essential to healthy family life (Giovanni, 1995). More specifically, a family is a system of two or more interacting persons who are related by ties of marriage, birth, or adoption or who have chosen to commit themselves to each other as a unit for the common purpose of promoting the physical, mental, emotional, social, cultural, and spiritual growth and development of each of its members (Pardeck & Yuen, 1997).

This definition is intended to be more inclusive than those traditionally used. It takes into consideration the nature, structure, and function of the family. As the fundamental or primary unit of a society, the family and its functions are intricately tied to the needs of the family as assessed by the family itself and the community or communities of which it is a member (Daly et al., 1995; Pardeck & Yuen, 1997).

In his discussion of community, William G. Brueggemann (1996) identifies family as more than a collection of individuals sharing a specific physical and psychological space. A family is a natural social system that has attributes of its own, an organized power structure, and assigned and ascribed roles for its members. A family has a set of rules and has developed intricate overt and covert forms of communication, elaborate ways of negotiating and problem solving that allow various tasks to be performed effectively. The relationship between members of a family is based primarily on a shared history, shared internalized perceptions and assumptions about the world, and a shared sense of purpose. Within this system, individuals are bound to one another by powerful, durable, reciprocal emotional attachments and loyalties that may fluctuate in intensity over time but persist over the lifetime of the family.

Health

The concept of *health* as used here is defined by the World Health Organization (cited in Giovanni, 1995). Philip R. Popple, Leslie Leighninger, and S. Parkinson (1996, p. 406) describe health as "a state of complete physical, mental, and social well-being and not merely the absence of disease or [pathology]." However, assessing health is more often discussed in terms of the absence of health or mortality and morbidity. In the concept of this chapter, health rather than illness gets primary focus.

Family Health

Family health is viewed as a state of holistic well-being for the family. It is manifested by the development of and continuous interaction among the physical, mental, emotional, social, cultural, and spiritual dimensions of the family (Pardeck & Yuen, 1997). Health care is designed to treat, prevent, and detect physical, mental, and social disfunctioning and to enhance people's physical and psychosocial well-being. The health care system includes educational and environmental facilities that help people prevent disease.

Community

Numerous discrete definitions of *community* are currently in use in social science literature. Although they are so diverse that no one definition or theory seems to capture their total essence, common to all of the definitions are concepts such as *space, people, interaction*, and *shared identity* (Netting, Kettner, & McMurtry, 1998, p. 104).

As with family, community consists of natural human associations based on ties of kinship, relationship, and shared experience in which individuals voluntarily attempt to provide meaning in their lives, meet needs, and accomplish personal goals. They share certain practices that define the community and those who are nurtured by it. Community almost always has a history defined in part by its past and its memory of its past that ''exists before individuals are born and which will continue after their death'' (Brueggemann, 1996, p. 110).

Mark S. Homan (1994) defines community as having a common connection that may be a place where members live, such as a city or a neighborhood; an activity, for example, a job; or a racial or ethnic identification, such as Native Americans. Communities may be made up of sets of smaller communities; that is, cities have different neighborhoods, universities have different colleges and departments, and softball leagues have different teams.

TYPES OF COMMUNITIES: FUNCTION, ROLE, AND RESPONSIBILITIES

William G. Brueggemann (1996, p. 110) identifies three kinds of community—modern, ontological or ''communities of meaning,'' and traditional—while others distinguish ways of categorizing community based on place or geographic locale, identification or interest, and personal network.

Global or world is another concept of community that is used in contemporary society to refer to the complicated arrangement of relationships among the world's people. This term focuses on relationships that transcend traditional geographical boundaries. Such relationships may be bound by various characteristics previously identified, in addition to concern for common issues and frequent communication (Netting et al., 1998).

Functional communities of identification and interest are formed when people come together around common issues. Commonalities may include racial and ethnic diversity, populations at risk, or those who have been victimized by social and economic injustice.

What Would a Healthy Community Look Like?

The social constructionist theoretical framework requires individuals belonging to a particular community to define and determine for themselves what they think constitutes a healthy community. However, several factors could be considered part of any healthy community:

1. *Individuals and families want to be a part of a community* as opposed to society placing or requiring one to be a part of a particular community because of race, ethnicity, sexual orientation, religion, or socioeconomic class. One example that pertains to a geographical community is the situation with public housing. Many of the families who live there do so because they feel they have to; they have no place else to go. These authors argue that one of the most critical features of a healthy community is that people "belong" who *want* to belong. Choice is essential.
2. *A safe environment* is one in which families feel safe from physical violence, governmental and environmental neglect and abuse, and economic exploitation.
3. *Access to quality health care* should not be dependent upon one's not living in an economically poor rural or inner-city community or not having a socially unacceptable disease such as AIDS.
4. *A low crime rate* is correlated with a safe environment—minority groups and low-income individuals who may already have the fewest resources should not also have the highest potential for victimization by crime.
5. *Low unemployment and underemployment rates* are necessary in order for families to meet their basic survival needs of food, shelter, clothes, and so forth, particularly in this time of welfare reform and greater conservatism, at least toward the poor.
6. *Good educational systems* are essential if families are to help their children develop into successful, interdependent, healthy adults.

7. *Sufficient, adequate, and safe housing* includes the concept of sufficient individual personal space and is required for families to be safe and healthy.
8. *Transportation* is correlated with employment and also may be with health care. Particularly for low-income families, good employment and health care are not located within their geographical communities. If individuals are to access these resources, transportation is a significant key.
9. *Low violence* includes violence both internal and external to families. in their neighborhoods and going to and from school or recreation, children need to grow up in environments that are free from violence. They should feel safe in these areas. They also need to be free of experiencing violence as the victims of abuse or of witnessing violence as a result of family abuse or battering.
10. *Adequate recreation and leisure* are as important to healthy individual, family, and community functioning as is work. Because individuals may have marginal status in society, it does not mean their need to play is any less than those of other communities.

THEORETICAL FRAMEWORK

The theoretical frameworks which John T. Pardeck and Francis K. O. Yuen (1997) identified as functional to the concept of community-centered family health are systems theory, ecological theory, and social constructionism. These theories provide a framework for understanding human behavior, its relationship, interrelatedness, and interaction in the social environment.

Ecological Theory

The ecological perspective sees the community as an organism that has boundaries and engages in transactional and reciprocal exchanges with the environment. The outcome of this exchange is a hemostatic balance in which the biosystem is held in equilibrium. A healthy social organism is one in which all of the different components fit together with one another and that has adapted to its environment.

Social Systems Theory

The social systems model adopts a structural/functional model of communities. A community is composed of a series of interrelated parts, each of which serves a specific function in the community structure. In other words, each component of a community exists for a purpose (Brueggemann, 1996).

Pardeck and Yuen (1997, p. 125) have cautioned others of the limitations of both the ecological perspective and social systems perspective. They argue that "sensitivity to the work of social constructionists may help practitioners understand the potential limitations of the systems and ecological approaches to practice, giving meaning to reality. The family health approach emphasizes the importance of considering the client's view of social reality when assessing a presenting problem."

In this regard, the authors of this chapter explore action theory as a conceptual framework for understanding critical dynamics of the community. They seek to provide a clear explanation of situational experiences that impact one's ability to think of an engaged community that has the capability of promoting health.

Action Theory

According to Brueggemann (1996), the action theory of social work reestablishes community as centering on the sentiments that unite people. It includes community as the arena in which humans find their identity as social beings who are active agents in the creation of social reality. B. L. Fenby (1991) states that action theory focuses on introspection, the reflective use of the self, and choices that are consistent with one's moral beliefs.

Brueggemann (1996) asserts that a sense of community exists because of values, sentiments, feelings of identification and commitment held in common by a collective of individuals. He further states that because of the significance of these factors, the concept of community is not confined to a boundary or geographic locality. For individuals that share mutual sentiments, common identity, and a sense of caring regardless of the locality, they can create a sense of community through the commonality of their bonds. This explanation of community provides a different approach to creating a community when it does not exist in the traditional sense.

Action theory offers an alternative for developing a nurturing environment that extends beyond a specific location that can contribute to the health and well-being of families. The implications for this theory provide individuals, groups, organizations, and communities with a different strategy for organizing themselves in a manner that promotes family health. Action theory embodies a constructionist perspective in that the social constructionist approach attempts to foster change by opening up new views of reality (Berg & De Jong, 1996).

According to Bill Lee and Wendy Weeks (1991, p. 223), the women's movement serves as a viable model to understanding action theory as it relates to the concept of community:

> Women's movement community organizing has had to build a community of women, (a different view of reality) because the structure of women's lives, more often than not, has mitigated against community. The emphasis by the women's movement on the "personal is political" has meant that the family and personal life have become targets for social action beliefs, values and sentiments held in common.

Another organization that has redefined its community is the American Association of Retired Persons (AARP). This organization came together around shared needs, values, and sentiments. Originally founded to address the health care needs of retired schoolteachers, AARP no longer serves only retired teachers but now includes in its membership any individual 50 years old and older who shares a variety of common sentiments. By working together and redefining themselves and their interest and concern about ageism, this organization has grown to become one of the most politically influential organizations in the country (American Association of Retired Persons, 1998).

Many constituent groups bound by shared beliefs, values, and common interest have the potential to compose various communities. These communities may or may not be defined by a geographic location, but they can aid in supporting family health. Another example includes Alcoholics Anonymous (AA) and Alanon. These communities are loosely united around self-identification, experiences, sentiments, and concern and caring for the recovering substance abuser. Such nontraditional communities nurture individuals and provide structure to their lives, resources, and the opportunity to meet on a regular basis. This collective sharing helps to facilitate recovery and the challenges that members face in their everyday lives. Although not geographically bounded, AA communities exist in most states throughout the country. In a real sense these groups can be said to promote community family health. These authors offer strategies and solutions based on similar approaches that address family health–centered community practice.

COMMUNITY CHANGE

Communities have continued to change for various reasons in society. Structural conditions have greatly influenced modern-day society. The largest impact on urban communities began with the industrial era in America. As the country shifted from an agricultural period to an industrial one, many previous rural residents migrated to cities seeking new jobs and higher wages. Many occupied overcrowded dwellings. Migration has historically been a part of urban life, especially in major cities like New York, Chicago, and Detroit.

The traditional ambience of communities—for example, ice cream and candy stores and people sitting on front porches watching their neighbors walk by—appears to be a time of the past. These were traditional communities.

Most scholars, regardless of their ideological perspective, agree that neighborhood community is a vital institution to urban democracy that determines how well urbanites adjust to their environment. Their disagreements lie in whether neighborhoods were constructed out of class or ethnic ties or whether transience prevented the formation of neighborhood communities (Jansson, 1994). These authors believe external factors such as transience and structural conditions in society, especially socioeconomic factors, helped to destabilize many traditional communities.

As more able families become more economically independent, they are able to move into communities that are less crowded. Many companies have relocated job opportunities to the suburbs. The poorest of the poor, especially those living in public housing; the working poor; and the homeless are temporarily stranded in communities that are gutted of many economic opportunities.

The urban evolution has been compounded by the recession years of the 1970s and the downsizing of corporate America in the 1980s and 1990s. This and other factors have created a mismatch of jobs and labor skills to meet the needs of a highly technological society. This places individuals and families at a disadvantage, leaving them in chronic states of poverty, a risk factor for many social problems and poor family health.

The retreat from social justice has helped to set more rigid cultural, social, and economic boundaries around many minority communities. To meet the challenge, the profession must not only be able to support community empowerment but also join the struggle for group self-determination (Rivera & Erlich, 1981). The new challenges of the twenty-first century involve constructing a power base for survival and opportunity for the last core of ethnical and racial minorities that are coming to the table; that is, African Americans, Hispanic/Latino, Asian Americans, and Native Americans. These and other minority group status members such as women, people with disabilities, and the elderly all want their inherent rights under the constitution which includes justice for all. According to Felix G. Rivera and John L. Erlich:

> One of the most pressing issues of the 1980s was the changing nature of ethnic minority communities as it affects community organizing and social work education. The changing and emerging communities are a result of the increase in the Black, Latino and Asian populations. Others include Pacific Islanders and especially the Indochinese refugees, Native Americans, and the continued oppression of these communities. These trends were true in the 1980s and are also true in the 1990s. (1981, p. 189)

These ethnic families are most often isolated from and/or denied economic opportunities to attain middle-class status. These communities are characterized by high rates of poverty, unemployment, families headed by women, out-of-wedlock pregnancy, and the crime rate. Some social scientists maintain that "the departure of substantial numbers of working- and middle-class people has removed an important social buffer as well as role models who had stressed the importance of education and of visible, steady employment" (Devore & Schlesinger, 1996, p. 66).

COMMUNITY FUNCTIONS

As indicated earlier, geographical communities generally are structured to perform particular functions for their members. Some social researchers advocate the position that to understand community requires the analysis of both structure and function together. "Structures such as schools, churches, or political entities are intertwined with functions such as teaching, providing leadership and advocating for change" (Netting et al., 1998, p. 109). The concept of geographical community means organization of social activities that affords people access to what is necessary for day-to-day living. A community may or may not have specific boundaries, but community is significant because it performs functions necessary for human survival.

Diverse ethnic group communities of meaning maintain, promote, and keep alive the heritage, religion, history, culture, and traditions of a people. Similarly, churches, temples, and synagogues are communities whose past rituals, traditions, and literature continue to inform modern-day people with a sense of fellowship and unity. Communities are not only a particular historical era, place, or time; they are also a component of the human condition. Because it seems deeply rooted in human nature, community can be seen as a universal phenomenon.

Although all individuals live in and identify to some extent with the community in which they live, Netting et al. (1998) maintain that some communities are seen as oppressive, restrictive, or even dangerous to the people who live there as well as to others who may live outside of the community.

Building on concepts developed in the 1970s, Netting et al. (1998) discuss community function as the framework for analysis. That source identified six functions that were performed by locality-relevant (geographical) communities: (a) production, distribution, and consumption; (b) socialization; (c) social control; (d) social participation; (e) mutual support; and (f) defense and communication.

Production, Distribution, and Consumption

The functions are designed to meet people's material needs, including the basic requirements such as food, clothing, shelter. People today are interdependent for basic needs as food, clothing, shelter, medical care, sanitation, employment, transportation, recreation, and other goods and services. The accepted medium of exchange is money. Thus money becomes an important factor in defining the limits of consumption and comes into consideration in most (if not all) community change efforts.

Socialization

Socialization pertains to the establishment of the prevailing norms, traditions, and values of those with whom people interact within a particular community. Socialization guides attitudinal development, and these attitudes and perceptions influence how people view themselves, others, and their interpersonal rights and responsibilities.

Social Control

Social control is the process by which community members ensure compliance with norms and values by establishing laws, rules, and regulations, and by ensuring their enforcement. Social control is the function performed by institutions representing various sectors such as government, education, religion, and social services.

Social Participation

Social participation includes interaction with others in community groups, associations, and organizations. Because people are assumed to need some form of outlet, they find it in local churches, civic organizations, and informal neighborhood groups. Understanding the opportunities and patterns of social participation for a target population is helpful in assessing the extent to which a community is meeting the needs of its members.

Mutual Support

Mutual support is the function that families, friends, neighbors, volunteers, and professionals carry out in communities when they care for those who are sick, unemployed, and distressed. Helping professions and government-sponsored programs developed in response to the inability of other social institutions to meet the mutual-support needs of community members. It is important to remember in U.S. society, mutual support functions may be undermined by a dominant value system that places a premium on rugged individualism. Communities may be considered "healthy" or "unhealthy," "functional" or "dysfunctional," and "competent" or "incompetent" based on their ability or inability to meet community needs. This may be particularly true for oppressed target populations within some community boundaries.

Defense and Communication

Since the 1970s, others have added defense and communication to the five earlier concepts and definitions. Defense is the way in which communities take care of and protect their members. This is particularly important for communities that are unsafe and dangerous. "Defended communities" are those that have to focus a great deal of effort on looking after their members (Netting et al., 1998, p. 110). Often this is the case in government housing projects and other low-income areas where community members must protect their families and children from illegal drug trafficking, gang violence, and other criminal elements. Other examples of defended communities may include those persons who are gay or lesbian, since there are groups within the larger society that may seek to do them harm. Similarly, people of color in various communities have had to support one another in defending themselves against the violence of racial or ethnic hatred.

Communication is a function that includes the use of a common language and symbols to express ideas. The communication function is a critical one in a community, especially language ability and "power to define" and "name." Examples of the communication function include the current debate over such issues as political correctness, English-only, and ebonics.

STRATEGIES AND SOLUTIONS

Community Health Practice

Direct social work practice in health care traces back to 1900, when City Hospital in Cleveland used outdoor relief workers to clear hospital wards of chronic patients, homeless Civil War veterans, and others who were considered "unwelcome boarders." Direct practice has historically emphasized face-to-face interactions with clients, families, and small groups. It borrows heavily from traditional methods of social casework and group work. Medical and clinical social work refer to direct practice in health care and reflect social work's historically close alliance with medical professionals in hospitals and clinical settings (Giovanni, 1995; Jansson, 1997; Popple et al., 1996).

Community or indirect social work practice in health care began around the turn of the century when social workers became involved in preventing and controlling epidemics and debilitating diseases. Efforts of Jane Adams, Grace Abbott, and other social workers in the Settlement House movement redirected professional attention to health prevention and the need for systemic change. These early social workers used community action to eradicate substandard housing, poor sanitation, inadequate nutrition, poverty, and other conditions contributing to ill health in families and communities. Their collective efforts provided the foundation to community organization as a discrete social work practice method. These efforts expanded health social work in the areas such as public health and prevention, primary care, rehabilitation, mental health, and long-term care.

Traditionally, community health practice has emphasized social work's discrete practice methods of community organization, policy practice, and administration (Ehrenreich, 1985; Giovanni, 1995). However, other researchers envisioned a much larger understanding of health that takes into account human relationships, community life, temperament, and financial circumstances. These individuals in the health field have consistently held to a much broader view of direct social work practice. This view, consistent with the concept of family health–centered community practice presented in this chapter, includes attention to families and social conditions that affect their health and the community well-being (Jansson, 1997).

The community arena has not been particularly well conceptualized; nor has it received the focus or articulation it needs in clinical social work theory. Social workers in all fields of practice must develop the knowledge and skills required to deal with environmental influences that affect the psychosocial functioning of families and communities (Rothman, Erlich, & Tropman, 1995).

What Are Potential Solutions?

Schools of social work must also look back to one of the most influential periods in history, the 1960s, when community organization helped reshape the face of the American people. Through looking back, the profession can begin to focus on methods and strategies that were effective. There is a need to revise and redefine old strategies, systems, and institutions and make them available, acceptable, accessible, affordable, and appropriate (Randal-David, 1989).

Let's refer to an earlier example in this chapter, in which AA is identified as a system that has developed a community of recovering individuals. These individuals have come together around shared identity, goals, and sentiments. Through the help and support that individuals provide to each other, a bond can be formed that serves as an ingredient for cementing a group. This movement began as a self-help movement and has grown to a point where there are currently self-help groups all across the country. Not only did AA create a nurturing environment for individuals; it became a community for recovering substance abusers.

The AA model and methodology also had a macroimpact in that it has been adopted by many new groups. Other groups modeled after AA include Gamblers Anonymous, Overeaters Anonymous, Parents Anonymous, Mothers Against Drunk Drivers, victims' groups, and many others.

Certainly the alcohol and substance abuse recovery of users impacts the health of individuals, families, and communities. If Alcoholics Anonymous chooses to redefine another aspect of its conceptual framework, it has the potential to organize chapters across the country into political action communities that address the issue of substances in communities at the local, state, and national levels. Through redefining its role among a community of recovering individuals, their numbers, clout, and methodology, clearly AA has the ingredients to promote and impact community change beyond the group or mezzo level.

It becomes reasonable to think that many of the strategies used by organizations such as the women's movement, AARP, Alcoholics Anonymous, and others could be utilized by individuals wishing to address some basic survival needs. In communities where a sense of community does not exist, a new community or alternative sense of community may need to be reconceptualized to meet and address common goals and interest.

Community Health

The health and economic vitality of its members and effective policy making are included among the needs of each community. As with families, when these needs are not adequately met, discomfort to members results, health problems develop, and community change needs to occur. Because we have concluded that communities function as systems, community change is seen as systems change. Community change is the process of producing modification or innovation in attitudes, policies, or practices in the community for the purpose of reducing or eliminating problems or providing for general improvement in the way needs are met (Homan, 1994; Segal & Brzuzy, 1998). This process enhances the quality of health of the family and their relationship among members. For the community that is having problems meeting its needs, there must be change before there can be a healthy community.

It is important that health care practices be more closely aligned with community expectations and needs as defined by the community. Families in minority communities, particularly African American and Native American, have a history of underutilization of existing health services. One indicator of this is an infant mortality rate among some minorities that is as much as two and a half times higher than those of the majority community. Hesitancy to pursue appropriate medical services has been attributed to "explicit acts of racial stereotyping of Black patients by White physicians, collusion among White-dominated health organizations to exclude Black physicians, and adoption by health providers of a White model of health services" (Green, 1995, p. 33).

The inhibiting of opinions and emotions, forced and false smiles contrived to assure the dominant group that they are not "angry," and the suppressed rage creates daily strain for many minorities living in the United States. African Americans, especially black men, suffer inordinately high levels of hypertension, an illness that reflects social as well as medical causes (Brown, 1995; Butler, 1994; Hacker, 1995).

A major challenge for family health is operationalizing the concept for practitioners, educators, and others. Although the concept is not new, operationalizing it is revolutionary in that it requires that the concept of health is connected to all social systems' functioning. This also includes biological, psychological, social, and economic issues related to holistic well-being (Daly et al., 1995). The case has to be made wherein a health relationship between individuals, families, groups, organizations, communities, and society are viewed as being interrelated. This requires a redefinition of the concept of health.

Let's refer to an earlier example. In order to further connect the case of substance abuse and family health, some basic questions must be asked:

1. Why do people produce drugs?
2. Why do people use drugs?
3. Why do people sell illegal drugs?
4. How do production, distribution, and use of drugs affect the health of U.S. families?
5. How do production, distribution, and use of drugs affect the health of communities?

It could be argued that questions 1 and 3 are related to structural conditions in society (e.g., economy, jobs, foreign policy). In terms of question 1, why people produce drugs, in many countries the production of hard drugs is a national commodity of the economy. Drugs are a lucrative economic market. Questions 2 and 4 are much more difficult to answer because they require an understanding of the biopsychosocial needs of users and the identification of the interrelationship between each and its impact on U.S. society.

People use drugs for various reasons. These are often associated with psychological and social factors such as peer pressure, emotional fulfillment, experimentation, exposure to substance abuse in the home, family distress, and numerous other reasons related to unhealthy family functioning. Another reason could be the glamorization of drug use through the portrayal of crime in the media.

Research indicates a correlation between substance abuse, incest, sexual abuse, and physical abuse. Since illegal drug use is so massive and has such a detrimental effect on families and communities, a decrease of drug flow into the country should be an immediate priority.

In 1983 a comprehensive economic analysis was conducted. The cost of alcohol problems in America was estimated to exceed $70 billion per year. An additional $44 billion in economic cost was attributed to drug problems. Alcohol is associated with nearly half of all deaths caused by motor vehicle crashes and fatal intentional injuries such as suicides and homicides. Victims are intoxicated in approximately one third of all homicides, drowning, and boat-related deaths (Department of Health and Human Services, 1990).

Substance abuse also presents problems for teenagers. Problems include school failure, early unwanted pregnancy, and delinquency. Abuse of alcohol and other drugs significantly increases the risk of transmitting the Human Immunodeficiency Virus (HIV), directly through the sharing of contaminated needles and through sexual contact with intravenous drug abusers. Alcohol is a principal contributor to cirrhosis and birth defects. Homeless alcohol abusers are at substantial increased risk of trauma, victimization, hypothermia, frostbite, and tuberculosis infection. Alcohol and other drugs may be, in many situations, both the cause and effect of homelessness.

The *Healthy People 2000* document (Department of Health and Human Services, 1990) further states that widespread substance abuse is having an enormous impact on the country. Almost every national opinion poll places alcohol and other drug problems as a priority concern, and the national efforts to prevent these problems have mobilized government, schools, communities, businesses, and families.

Although many Americans are intolerant of the use of illicit drugs and misuse of alcohol, there does not appear to be the same level of intolerance for the biopsychosocial and economic needs of users. The supply and demand side of the drug trade is directly interrelated to family health and community well-being.

Answering these questions will serve a vital role in helping practitioners recognize the levels of interventions that are required to address the gravity of this social problem. The issue of substance abuse is so massive that interventions at all social levels are required. It is the opinion of the authors that no single solution can be effective without attacking the problem from top to bottom. However, most practitioners will find themselves addressing the problem at the direct service level.

If we start at the individual client level of the substance abuse scenario, the abuser becomes the focal system. For example, social work practitioners will have to:

1. Be trained to detect the potential use of substances among abusers.
2. Conduct a biopsychosocial assessment of the client to assess the types of interventions that will be used and willingness of the client to cooperate.
3. Assess the impact of the abuse on the family health of its members.
4. Conduct subsequent assessments on all members of the family to determine the impact of the substance abuse on the unit.
5. Develop an intervention and treatment plan in partnership with all members that includes addressing the biopsychosocial, cultural, and spiritual needs of the family.
6. Monitor the progress of all family members.
7. Evaluate the progress of all family members.

Agencies and organizations that employ social workers have to also be invested in redefining family and health. Alcohol and drug abuse are used in this material as just one example of a problem that affects the health of the community. There are many such social problems.

Many social welfare organizations and agencies that work with families recognize that the problem of a particular member has direct implications for other members that can affect their health and well-being.

Many also recognize that other family members may have problems that are separate from the focal client system. This will require administrators, staff, and social workers to identify the connections between holistic health and well-being for the families that the agency serves. Community priorities should bring the community health practitioner to a closer view of the community's perception of reality. Issues such as good jobs and employment are intricately linked to good health (Daly et al., 1995; Saleebey, 1994). Practitioners will have to:

1. Examine the impact of designing and redesigning the ways that organizations provide family health services.
2. Identify how holistic state of well-being and family health can be promoted and implemented within the agency.
3. Consult with members to clarify what family health means to each family.
4. Appropriately educate the work force.
5. Conduct an assessment of family health–related cases within the organization.
6. Determine what resources are available to make transitions in service from a client focus system to a family health focus system.
7. Examine whether the agency needs to redesign its tools and instruments for collecting data.

At the community level the social work practitioner will work with individuals, groups, and organizations. The practitioner's role will be slightly different:

1. Conduct a needs assessment with (not for) the community about knowledge, attitude, and practices of substance abuse issues in the community.
2. Identify partners who are willing to take action regarding substance abuse.
3. Be willing to learn from community members and educate members and organizations about substance abuse and its impact on family health.
4. Identify with the community regarding its priorities pertain-

ing to family health and interrelated biopsychosocial issues concerning substance abuse.

5. Identify resources and strengths currently available or in process of development that will meet the needs of community members.
6. Identify gaps in services.
7. Examine and identify how their programs and services relate to family health.
8. Form coalitions or partnerships to facilitate closing gaps in services for families in the community in order to address the biopsychosocial, economic, cultural, and spiritual needs of families.
9. Design a plan or intervention with the community.
10. Identify resources for the plan.
11. Coordinate the implementation of the plan.
12. Monitor and evaluate the plan.
13. For communities of color, articulate family health needs and intervention plans within the context of their cultural environment.

Social Workers' Role

The perceptions and perspectives of social workers should not take precedence over the community's ability to problem-solve or the critical components that they bring in the interpretation of their reality (Brueggemann, 1996). For example, from a public health perspective practitioners looking at public health data may decide to conduct health promotion programs in poor minority communities. They are convinced this is needed because staggering health statistics validate their claim. In addition, they are witnessing trends in their clinics and facilities that mirror state and national trends. Health practitioners are convinced that health promotion activities will be beneficial to the community. Who could argue with this idea, knowing that African Americans and other minorities suffer and die disproportionately from preventable diseases?

Social workers must be aware of how persons will be affected by change, define, and perceive their communities. They should understand perspectives that may be different from their own worldview, recognize the assumptions and values that undergird these views, and consider how differing perspectives can influence change opportunities (Saleebey, 1994). It is also significant to remember that persons within the same community may differ in their perspectives or definition of what community is and what changes are needed.

Often viewed as networks or webs of formal or informal resources, relationships and what they mean to a person's "sense of community" are important for social workers to recognize, respect, and understand (Daly et al., 1995). If people find their "sense of community" through disparate, scattered relationships that do not interface, it may be difficult to mobilize them to want to address a local community need.

Personal networks or membership in multiple communities is another strategy for promoting healthy families and communities. In a complex society people establish their own array of relationships based on both place and nonplace. Belonging to multiple communities contributes toward individual, family, and community development. It is a way in which individuals and families grow, develop, and are actualized. With multiple communities, families have access to more and improved information, financial resources, employment, and social networks. Individuals gain more from each of the multiple communities with whom they are associated and also contribute more in the same manner. Specific communities with whom the individual or family is associated change and keep pace with the lifespan of the individual and the family.

SUMMARY AND CONCLUSION

Problems and needs can often be addressed more effectively by dealing with them collectively rather than individually. Enfranchisement and empowerment can be significant vehicles for the creation of healthy communities when there is awareness, understanding, and action. The goal of becoming members of multiple communities is self-actualization through healthy family and community function.

Family health is interconnected to society. Everyone is born, stays well or gets sick, and dies. Health is a universal thread that is woven into a physiological structure impacted by psychosocial and spiritual factors. For organizations and communities that serve families, this means they will need to assess whether their organizations are capable of providing or attaining holistic services for their clients. Obtaining additional training may be required to provide knowledge about family health issues. At the community level, needs assessments will have to be conducted with the community to determine what is needed. Family health practitioners will have to train, be educated, and partner with communities.

Each social group, organization, and community must acknowledge health as a critical element of social well-being. Last but not least, each social entity must become health promoters in order to address family health. Many examples have been provided that serve as guides for redefining community. The challenge for communities is to take advantage of the opportunities they have to promote family health. Just as it takes a village to raise a child, it takes a community to promote family health.

REFERENCES

American Association of Retired Persons (AARP). (1998). *About AARP membership.* [Online]. Available: http://www.aarp.org/who.html.

Berg, I. K., & De Jong, P. (1996). Solutions—Building conversations: Co-constructing a sense of competence with clients. *Journal of Contemporary Human Services, 77*(6), 376.

Brown, C. (1995). Empowerment in social work practice with older women. *Social Work, 40*, 359–364.

Brueggemann, W. (1996). *The practice of macro social work.* Chicago: Nelson-Hall.

Butler, L. (1994). *African American women's advanced educational attainment: Enabling and restricting factors.* Unpublished doctoral dissertation, Ohio State University, Columbus.

Daly, A., Jennings, J., Beckett, J., & Leashore, B. (1995). Effective coping strategies of African Americans. *Social Work, 40*, 240–248.

Department of Health and Human Services. (1990). *Healthy people 2000: National health promotion and disease prevention objectives* (No. PHS 91-50212). Washington, DC: Government Printing Office.

Devore, W., & Schlesinger, E. (1996). *Ethnic-sensitive social work practice.* Boston: Allyn and Bacon.

Ehrenreich, J. (1985). *The altruistic imagination: A history of social work and social policy in the United States.* Ithaca, NY: Cornell University Press.

Fenby, B. L. (1991). Feminist theory, critical theory and management's romance with the technical. *Affilia, 6*(1), 20.

Floyd, H. H. (1980). Family health policy formation: A problematic definitional process. *Journal of Sociology and Social Welfare, 7*(4), 533.

Giovanni, J. (1995). Childhood. In *Encyclopedia of social work* (19th ed., pp. 433–441). Washington, DC: National Association of Social Work.

Green, J. (1995). *Cultural awareness in the human services: A multi-ethnic approach.* Boston: Allyn and Bacon.

Hacker, A. (1995). *Two nations: Black and white, separate, hostile, unequal.* New York: Ballantine Books.

Homan, M. (1994). *Promoting community change: Making it happen in the real world.* Pacific Grove, CA: Brooks/Cole.

Jansson, B. (1994). *Social policy: From theory to policy practice.* Pacific Grove, CA: Brooks/Cole.

Jansson, B. (1997). *The reluctant welfare state.* Pacific Grove, CA: Brooks/Cole.

Lee, B., & Weeks, W. (1991). Social action theory and the women's movement: An analysis of assumptions. *Community Development Journal, 26*(3), 221–226.

Netting, E., Kettner, P., & McMurtry, S. (1998). *Social work macro practice.* New York: Longman.

Pardeck, J. T., & Yuen, F. K. O. (1997). A family health approach to social work. *Family Therapy, 2*(24), 115–128.

Popple, P., Leighninger, L., & Parkinson, S. (1996). *Social work, social welfare, and American society.* Boston: Allyn and Bacon.

Randal-David, E. (1989). *Strategies for working with minority communities.* Bethesda, MD: U.S. Department of Health and Human Services (MCH 113793), Bureau of Maternal and Child Health and Resources Development, Brown Gray School of Medicine.

Rivera, F. G., & Erlich, J. L. (1981). Neo-Gemeinshaft minority communities: Implications for community organization in the United States. *Community Development Journal, 16*(3), 189–224.

Rothman, J., Erlich, J., & Tropman, J. (1995). *Strategies of community intervention.* Itasca, IL: F. E. Peacock.

Saleebey, D. (1994). Culture, theory, and narrative: The intersection of meaning in practice. *Social Work, 39*, 351–359.

Segal, E., & Brzuzy, S. (1998). *Social welfare policy, programs, and practice.* Itasca, IL: F. E. Peacock.

Index

About the Editors and Contributors

THE EDITORS

JOHN T. PARDECK is professor of social work in the School of Social Work at Southwest Missouri State University. He received his M.S.W. and Ph.D. in social work from St. Louis University. Pardeck has published numerous articles in academic and professional journals. His most recent books include *Social Work Practice: An Ecological Approach* (1996, Auburn House), *Reassessing Social Work Practice with Children* with Martha J. Markward (1997, Gordon and Breach Science Publishers), and *Social Work After the Americans with Disabilities Act: New Challenges and Opportunities for Social Services Professionals* (1998, Auburn House). Pardeck is a licensed clinical social worker and a member of the Academy of Certified Social Workers.

FRANCIS K. O. YUEN is an assistant professor for the School of Social Work at Southwest Missouri State University. He received his M.S.W. and D.S.W. from the University of Alabama, Tuscaloosa. He has many years of direct practice, program development, and agency management experience. In the past several years, he has developed four federally funded demonstration projects for various ethnic minority populations on family, health, and public health issues. His most recent family health–related publications include two articles: ''A Family Health Approach to Social Work Practice,'' with J. T. Pardeck, and ''Social Work Assessment and Intervention Through Family Health Practice'' with J. T. Pardeck, J. Daley, and C. Hawkins. His research interests focus on families in transition, substance abuse, violence, personal epistemology, diversity, management, and evaluation. He is also a member of the Academy of Certified Social Workers.

THE CONTRIBUTORS

Lola M. Butler, PhD, MSW.
Assistant Professor, School of Social Work,
Southwest Missouri State University, Springfield, MO 65804

Karen A. Callaghan, PhD.
Professor and Chair, Department of Sociology,
Barry University, Miami, FL 33161

James G. Daley, PhD, MSW.
Assistant Professor, School of Social Work,
Southwest Missouri State University, Springfield, MO 65804

Diane Elliott, MSSA.
Instructor, School of Social Work,
Southwest Missouri State University, Springfield, MO 65804

Catherine L. Hawkins, MSW, LCSW.
Director of Field Education, School of Social Work,
Southwest Missouri State University, Springfield, MO 65804

Mary Ann Jennings, PhD, MSSW.
Assistant Professor, School of Social Work,
Southwest Missouri State University, Springfield, MO 65804

Joan C. McClennen, PhD, MSW.
Assistant Professor, School of Social Work,
Southwest Missouri State University, Springfield, MO 65804

John T. Murphy, PhD.
Professor, Department of Sociology,
University of Miami, Coral Gables, FL 33124

John T. Pardeck, PhD, MSW.
Professor, School of Social Work,
Southwest Missouri State University, Springfield, MO 65804

Gregory J. Skibinski, PhD, MSW.
Associate Professor, School of Social Work,
Southwest Missouri State University, Springfield, MO 65804

Dee K. Vernberg, PhD.
Visiting Assistant Professor, Communication Studies,
The University of Kansas, Lawrence, KS 66045

Francis K. O. Yuen, DSW, MSW.
Assistant Professor, School of Social Work,
Southwest Missouri State University, Springfield, MO 65804